MEDITERRANEAN DIET COOKBOOK FOR BEGINNERS

130 Recipes Easy to Cook to Stay Fit and Follow a Healthy Eating Every Day.
7 Day Meal plan Included

Jennifer Skyman

TABLE OF CONTENTS

TABLE OF CONTENTS

TABLE OF CONTENTS

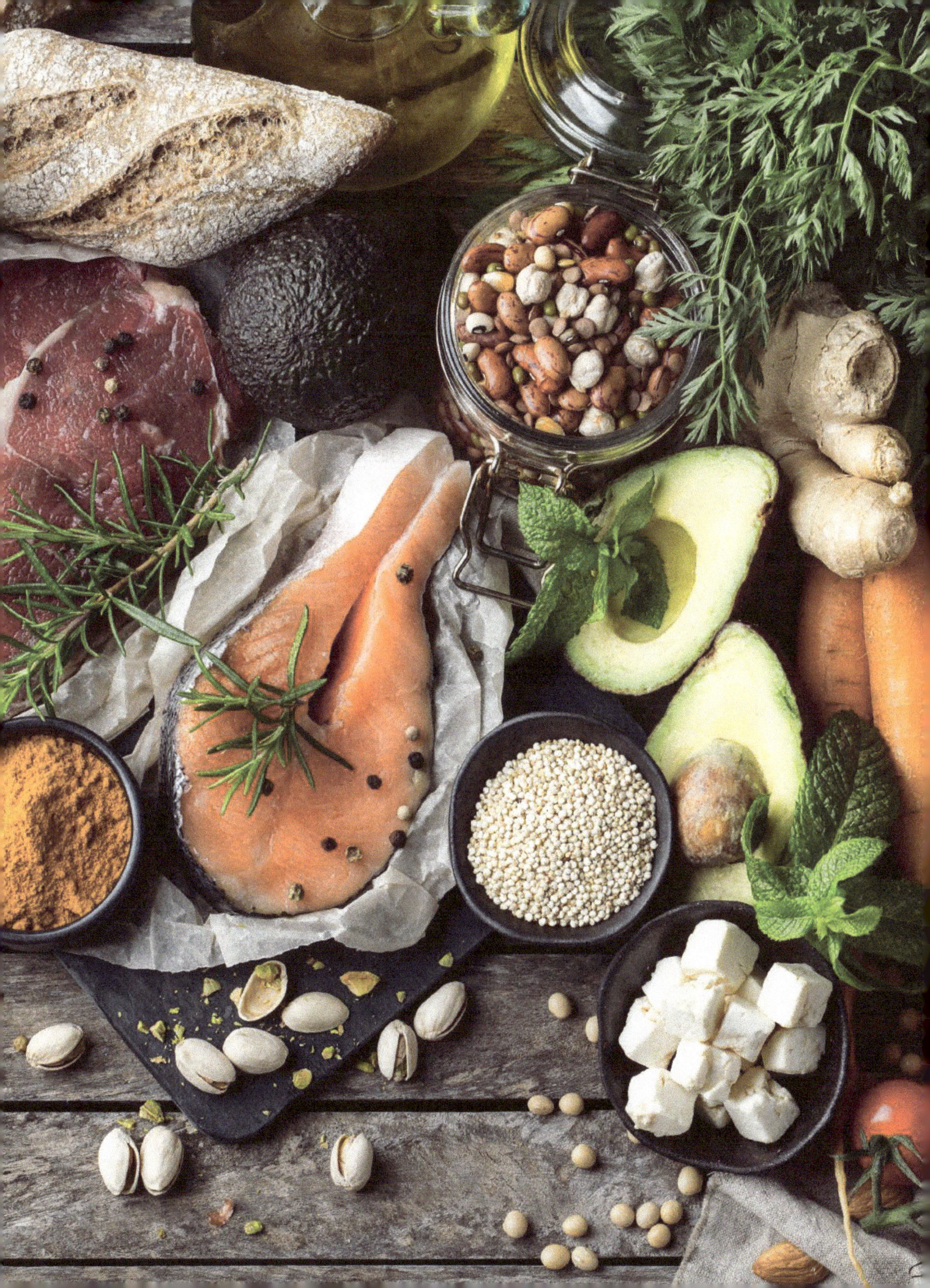

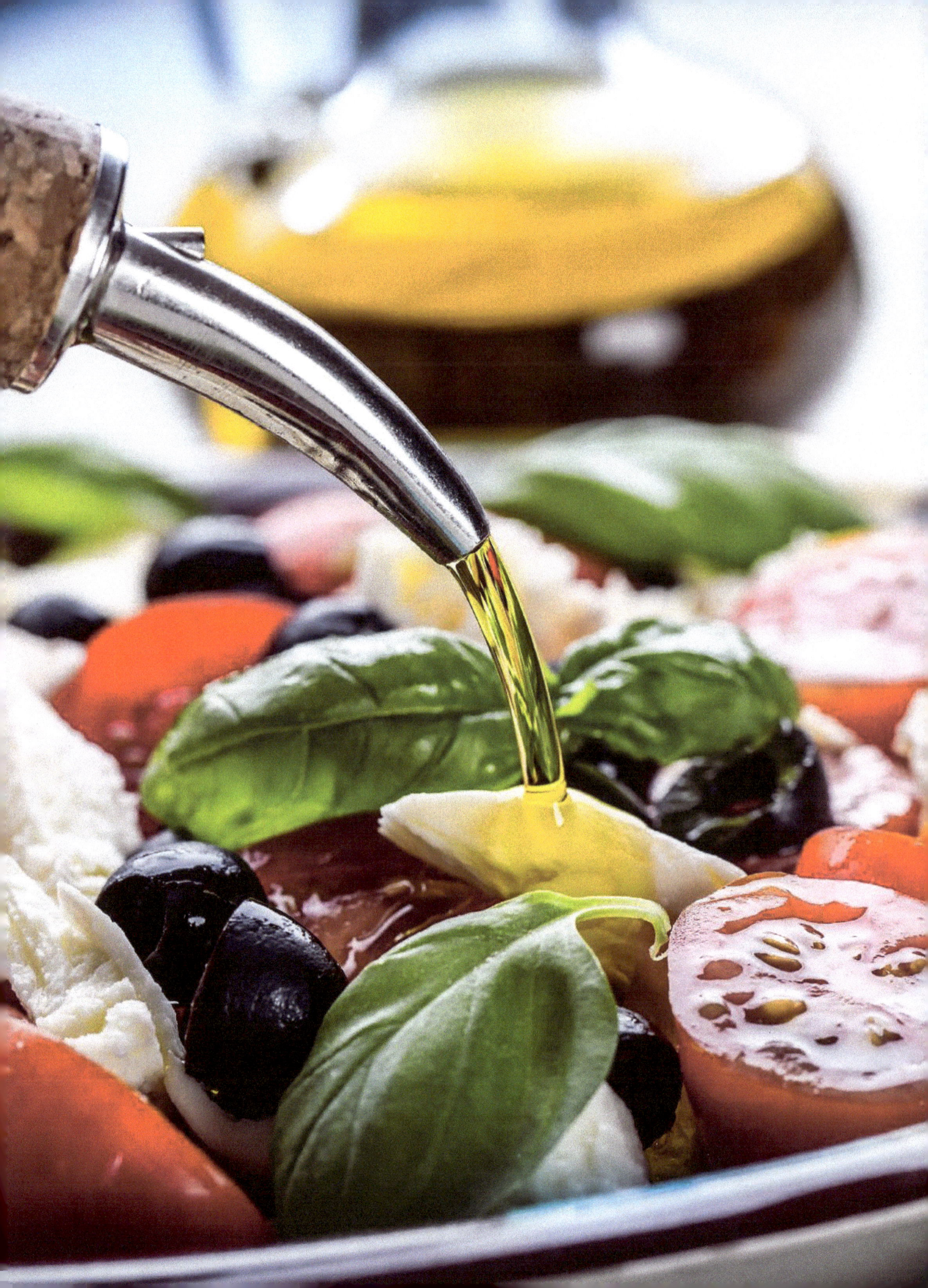

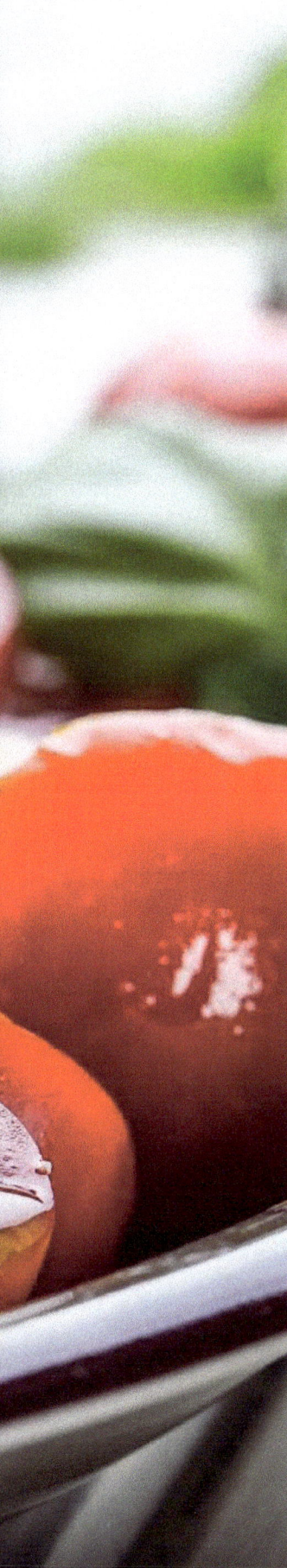

INTRODUCTION

Congratulations on purchasing the Mediterranean Diet Cookbook for Beginners: 130 Recipes Easy to Cook to Stay Fit and Follow a Healthy Eating Every Day. 7 Day Meal Plan Included

The following chapters will include batches of recipes including, delicious pork, seafood, poultry, lamb, beans, quinoa, various pizzas, flatbread options, and so many more delicious and healthy dishes. You can enjoy delightful fruit cups, yogurt dishes, and delicious snacking and dessert choices.

The Mediterranean Plan is built upon healthy fats as well as plant-based foods.

Since the plan does not eliminate entire food groups, it is believed you should not have any problems complying with it in the long term. Let's get started with the foods you should avoid while using the Mediterranean program. Remove these from your dieting Ingredients:

• **Processed Meat Products:** Processed sausages, bacon, Hot dogs, etc.

• **Refined Grains:** White bread and pasta made with refined wheat

• **Added Sugar:** Candy ice cream, regular soda, plus many others.

• **Refined Oils:** Soybean, canola, cottonseed, etc.

• **Red Meats:** (Limit to once each week)

You also achieve many benefits from the spices used on the dieting plan including, anise, bay leaves, basil, black pepper, cayenne pepper, ground chia seeds, cloves, cumin, and fennel. Ginger, garlic, marjoram, mint, oregano, parsley, sage, rosemary, and thyme also make excellent spice options. For a complete rundown of the listing, check the website at www.health.clevelandclinic.org. The calorie counts vary for each person, ranging from 1600 to 2400 range for women, and 2,000 up to 2,400 for men. Your meal plan has been left open for you to add the final snacks or other items you want to add to your delicious menu plan.

Now, you have the basics of the Mediterranean way of eating, let's learn how to prepare the delicious dishes!

1. MEDITERRANEAN BREAKFAST DISHES

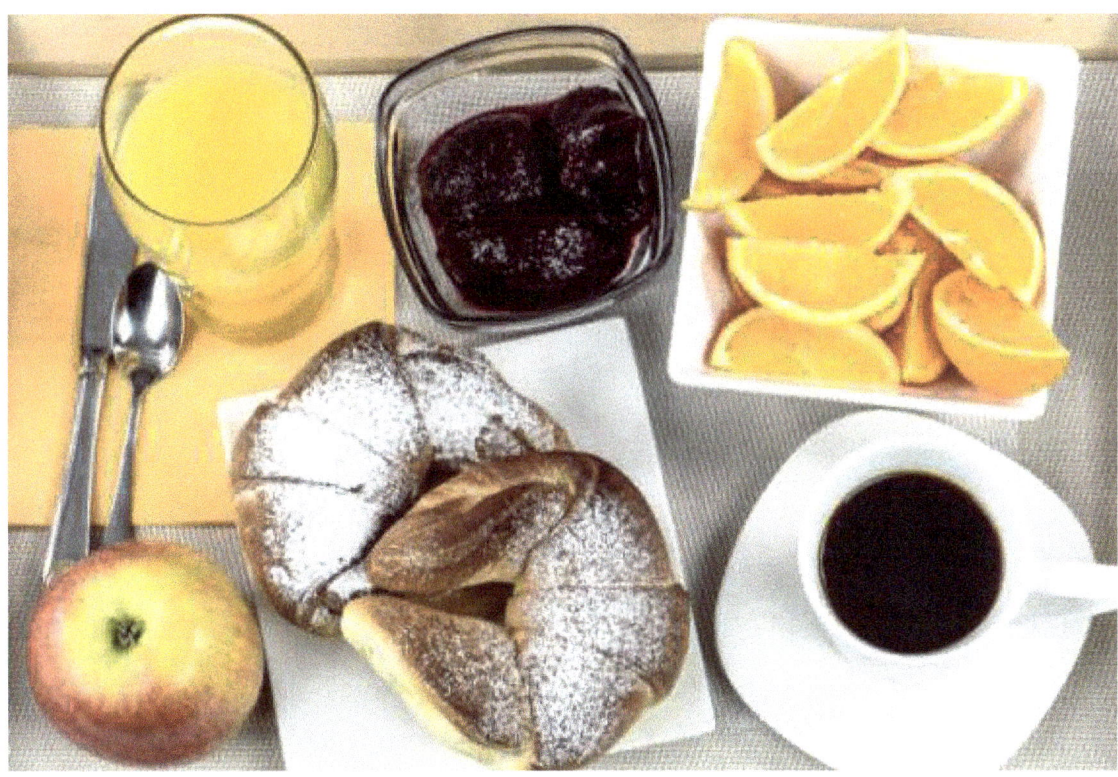

These delightful breakfast dishes will get your day started with its delicious and healthy Ingredients.

1.BAKED RICOTTA & PEARS

PREPARATION AND COOKINGTIME
30 MINUTES

SERVING
4 PEOPLE

INGREDIENTS

- **White whole wheat flour (.25 cup)**
- **Sugar (1 tbsp.)**
- **Nutmeg (.25 tsp.)**
- **Ricotta cheese - whole-milk (16 oz. container)**
- **Large eggs (2)**
- **Diced pear (1)**
- **Water (2 tbsp.)**
- **Vanilla extract (1 tsp.)**
- **Honey (1 tbsp.)**
- **Also Needed: 4 - 6 oz. ramekins**

DIRECTIONS

1. Warm the oven at 400° Fahrenheit.
2. Lightly spritz the ramekins with a cooking oil spray.
3. Whisk the flour, nutmeg, sugar, vanilla, eggs, and the ricotta together in a large mixing container.
4. Spoon the fixings into the dishes. Bake them for 20 to 25 minutes or until they're firm and set. Transfer them to the countertop and wait for them to cool.
5. In a saucepan, using the medium temperature setting, toss the cored and diced pear into the water for about ten minutes until it's slightly softened.
6. Take the pan from the burner and stir in the honey.
7. Serve the ricotta ramekins with the warm pear when it's ready.

Nutritions: *Calories: 312 Protein: 17 grams Fat: 17 grams*

2. CHEF JOHN'S POACHED EGG SPECIAL

PREPARATION AND COOKINGTIME
25 MINUTES

SERVING
2 PEOPLE

INGREDIENTS

- **Champagne vinegar (1 tsp.)**
- **Salt (.5 tsp.)**
- **Fresh eggs (2)**

DIRECTIONS

1. Pour cold water into a saucepan and wait for it to boil using the medium heat temperature setting. Stir in the salt and vinegar.
2. Break each of the eggs into a ramekin. Place it close to the water and slide it out of the dish. Simmer the egg to poaching until it's set.
3. Transfer the egg out of the pan using a slotted spoon (Continue cooking until the yolk is runny and the white is cooked, or about six minutes.)
4. Prepare a container with ice water. Transfer the eggs from the pan to the bowl of ice water (It slows and stops the cooking process.)
5. Place them onto a paper-lined plate and serve.

Nutritions: *Calories: 72 Protein: 6.3 grams Fat: 5 grams*

3. EGG WHITE SCRAMBLE WITH CHERRY TOMATOES & SPINACH

PREPARATION AND COOKINGTIME
8-10 MINUTES

SERVING
4 PEOPLE

INGREDIENTS

- **Olive oil (1 tbsp.)**
- **Eggs (1 whole) & Egg whites (10)**
- **Black pepper (.25 tsp.)**
- **Salt (.5 tsp.)**
- **Minced garlic clove (1)**
- **Halved cherry tomatoes (2 cups)**
- **Packed fresh baby spinach (2 cups)**
- **Light cream or Half & Half (.5 cup)**
- **Finely grated parmesan cheese (.25 cup)**

DIRECTIONS

1. Whisk the eggs, pepper, salt, and milk.
2. Prepare a skillet using the med-high temperature setting.
3. Toss in the garlic when the pan is hot to sauté for approximately 30 seconds.
4. Pour in the tomatoes and spinach, and continue to sauté it for one additional minute. The tomatoes should be softened, and the spinach wilted.
5. Add the egg mixture into the pan using the medium heat setting. Fold the egg gently as it cooks for about two to three minutes.
6. Remove from the burner, and sprinkle with a sprinkle of cheese.

Nutritions: *Calories: 142 Protein: 15 grams Fat: 2 grams*

4. FETA - AVOCADO & MASHED CHICKPEA TOAST

PREPARATION AND COOKINGTIME
15 MINUTES

SERVING
4 PEOPLE

INGREDIENTS

- **Chickpeas (15 oz. can)**
- **Diced feta cheese (2 oz. - .5 cup)**
- **Pitted avocado (1)**
- **Fresh juice: Lemon (2 tsp.) or orange (1 tbsp.)**
- **Black pepper (.5 tsp.)**
- **Honey (2 tsp.)**
- **Multigrain toast (4 slices)**

DIRECTIONS

1. Toast the bread. Drain the chickpeas in a colander. Scoop the avocado flesh into the bowl.
2. Use a large fork/potato masher to mash them until the mix is spreadable.
3. Pour in the lemon juice, pepper, and the feta.
4. Combine and divide onto the four slices of toast.
5. Drizzle using the honey and serve.

Nutritions: *Calories: 337 Protein: 13 grams Fat: 13 grams*

5. FETA FRITTATA

PREPARATION AND COOKINGTIME
25 MINUTES

SERVING
2 PEOPLE

INGREDIENTS

- **Garlic (1 small clove)**
- **Green onion (1)**
- **Large eggs (2)**
- **Egg substitute (.5 cup)**
- **Crumbled feta cheese - divided (4 tbsp.)**
- **Plum tomato (.33 cup)**
- **Avocado slices (4 thin)**
- **Reduced-fat sour cream (2 tbsp.)**
- **Also Needed: 6-inch skillet**

DIRECTIONS

1. Thinly slice/mince the onion, garlic, and tomato. Peel the avocado before slicing.
2. Heat the pan using the medium temperature setting and spritz it with cooking oil.
3. Whisk the egg substitute, eggs, and three tablespoons of the feta cheese.
4. Add the egg mixture into the pan. Cover and simmer for four to six minutes.
5. Sprinkle it using the rest of the feta cheese and tomato. Cover and continue cooking until the eggs are set or about two to three more minutes.
6. Wait for about five minutes before cutting it into halves.
7. Serve with the avocado and sour cream.

Nutritions: *Protein: 17 grams Fat: 12 grams Calories: 203*

6. FETA & QUINOA EGG MUFFINS

PREPARATION AND COOKINGTIME
45-50 MINUTES

SERVING
12 PEOPLE

INGREDIENTS

- **Cooked quinoa (1 cup)**
- **Chopped baby spinach (2 cups)**
- **Kalamata olives (.5 cup)**
- **Tomatoes (1 cup)**
- **White onion (.5 cup)**
- **Fresh oregano (1 tbsp.)**
- **Salt (.5 tsp.)**
- **Olive oil (2 tsp.+ more for coating pans)**
- **Eggs (8)**
- **Crumbled feta cheese (1 cup)**
- **Also Needed: 12-cup muffin tin**

DIRECTIONS

1. Heat the oven to reach 350° Fahrenheit.
2. Lightly grease the muffin tray cups with a spritz of cooking oil.
3. Prepare a skillet using the medium temperature setting and add the oil. When it's hot, toss in the onions to sauté for two minutes.
4. Dump the tomatoes into the skillet and sauté for one minute. Fold in the spinach and continue cooking until the leaves have wilted (1 min.).
5. Transfer the pot to the countertop and add the oregano and olives. Set it aside.
6. Crack the eggs into a mixing bowl, using an immersion stick blender to mix them thoroughly. Add the cooked veggies in with the rest of the fixings.
7. Stir until it's combined and scoop the mixture into the greased muffin cups.
8. Set the timer to bake the muffins for 30 minutes until browned, and the muffins are set.
9. Cool for about ten minutes.

Nutritions: *Calories: 113 Protein: 7 grams Fat: 7 grams*

7. 5-MINUTE HEIRLOOM TOMATO & CUCUMBER TOAST

PREPARATION AND COOKINGTIME
6-10 MINUTES

SERVING
1 PEOPLE

INGREDIENTS

- **Heirloom tomato (1 small)**
- **Persian cucumber (1)**
- **Olive oil (1 tsp.)**
- **Oregano (1 pinch)**
- **Kosher salt and pepper (as desired)**
- **Low-fat whipped cream cheese (2 tsp.)**
- **Trader Joe's Whole Grain Crispbread or your choice (2 pieces)**
- **Balsamic glaze (1 tsp.)**

DIRECTIONS

1. Dice the cucumber and tomato. Combine all of the fixings except for the cream cheese.
2. Smear the cheese on the bread, and add the mixture (step 1).
3. Top it off with the balsamic glaze and serve.

Nutritions: *Protein: 3 grams Fat: 8 grams Calories: 177*

8. FRUIT BULGUR BREAKFAST BOWLS

PREPARATION AND COOKINGTIME
20 MINUTES

SERVING
6 PEOPLE

INGREDIENTS

- **2% milk (2 cups)**
- **Uncooked bulgur (1.5 cups)**
- **Water (1 cup)**
- **Cinnamon (.5 tsp.)**
- **Frozen/fresh pitted dark sweet cherries (2 cups)**
- **Dried/fresh chopped figs (8)**
- **Chopped almonds (.5 cup)**

DIRECTIONS

1. Combine the cinnamon, water, milk, and the bulgur.
2. Stir once and bring to a boil. Put a top on the pot. Reduce the temperature setting to med-low.
3. Continue cooking until the liquid is absorbed (approx.10 min.).
4. Extinguish the flame, but leave the pan on the stove and stir in the cherries (frozen or thawed), almonds, and figs.
5. Stir well to thaw the cherries and hydrate the figs. Stir in the mint, and scoop into serving bowls.
6. Serve with warm milk or serve it chilled to your liking.

Nutritions: *Protein: 9 grams Fat: 6 grams Calories: 301*

9. HAM & EGG CUPS

PREPARATION AND COOKINGTIME
30 MINUTES

SERVING
8 PEOPLE

INGREDIENTS

- **Cooked ham - deli-style (8 thin slices)**
- **Mozzarella cheese (.25 cups/1 oz.)**
- **Eggs (8)**
- **Optional: Basil (8 tsp.)**
- **Black pepper (to taste)**
- **Grape or cherry tomatoes (6/as desired)**
- **Also Needed: Muffin tin (8-count)**

DIRECTIONS

1. Program the oven setting to 350° Fahrenheit. Coat the muffin tin cups with the spray.
2. Press the ham slice into the bottom and add the cheese to each of the prepared cups. Break an egg into the cup and sprinkle with the pepper. Add the pesto, if using. Slice the tomatoes into halves and place them on each of the cups.
3. Bake them for 18 to 20 minutes. The egg whites should be set, similar to a regular poached egg. Leave them in the cups for three to five minutes. Then, carefully take the cups out of the tin and serve.

Nutritions: *Calories: 145 Protein: 11 grams Fat: 10 grams*

10. 'HUEVOS' RANCHEROS

PREPARATION AND COOKINGTIME
15 MINUTES

SERVING
6 PEOPLE

INGREDIENTS

- **Salsa - ex. Old El Paso (16 oz. jar)**
- **Eggs (6)**
- **Flour tortillas/soft tacos (6-inch)**
- **Shredded cheese (.75 cup)**
- **Also Needed: 10-inch skillet**

DIRECTIONS

1. Heat the salsa until it's bubbly. Gently crack the eggs into the skillet.
2. Place a top on the pot and simmer using the med-low temperature setting for six to seven minutes. The eggs should be thoroughly cooked.
3. Warm the tortillas and serve using a sprinkle of cheese.
4. Spoon one egg onto each of the salsa filled tortillas and serve.

Nutritions: *Calories: 240 Protein: 11 grams Fat: 12 grams*

11. MARINARA EGGS WITH PARSLEY - GLUTEN-FREE

PREPARATION AND COOKINGTIME
20 MINUTES

SERVING
6 PEOPLE

INGREDIENTS

- **Olive oil (1 tbsp.)**
- **Eggs (6 large)**
- **Medium onion (half of 1 or 1 cup)**
- **Garlic (2 cloves or 1 tsp.)**
- **Diced tomatoes - undrained - no-salt-added (2 - 14.5 oz. cans)**
- **Chopped Italian fresh flat-leaf parsley (.5 cup)**
- **Optional: Crusty Italian bread with grated parmesan or Romano cheese**

DIRECTIONS

1. Heat a skillet using the med-high temperature setting. Add the oil.
2. Dice and toss the onions into the skillet. Sauté them for about five minutes. Stir occasionally and fold in the minced garlic, continuing to stir it for another minute.
3. Pour in the tomatoes with the juices into the pan and let it simmer until bubbling or for two to three minutes. Crack an egg into a coffee mug.
4. Once the tomatoes are boiling, lower the heat to medium. Use the spoon to make six indentions in the tomato mixture.
5. Add the egg to one of the slots and continue until you've used all of the eggs.
6. Place a top on the pot and cook for six to seven minutes or until done.
7. Garnish them with the parsley and serve with bread and grated cheese to your liking.

Nutritions: Calories: 122 Protein: 7 grams Fat: 7 grams

12. NUTTY ORANGE POLENTA

PREPARATION AND COOKINGTIME
15 MINUTES

SERVING
6 PEOPLE

INGREDIENTS

- **Plain polenta (2- 18-oz. tubes)**
- **2% milk - divided (2.25 - 2.5 cups)**
- **Oranges (2)**
- **Pecans (.5 cup)**
- **2% Plain Greek yogurt (.25 cup)**
- **Honey (8 tsp.)**

DIRECTIONS

1. Slice the polenta into rounds and place in a microwavable dish to heat for 45 seconds.
2. Prepare a pot using the medium heat setting and add the polenta. Mash it until it's roughly mashed.
3. In a microwavable dish, pour in the milk and heat it for one minute.
4. Pour two cups of warm milk into the pot with the polenta and whisk it thoroughly.
5. Add in milk a few tablespoons at a time until it's the way you like it. Let the mixture cook slowly for about five minutes. Take the pan off of the burner.
6. Peel and chop the onions and pecans.
7. Serve and garnish them with the oranges, pecans, honey, and yogurt before serving.

Nutritions: *Calories: 234 Protein: 3 grams Fat: 7 grams*

13. PEANUT BUTTER & BANANA GREEK YOGURT BOWL

PREPARATION AND COOKINGTIME
5 MINUTES

SERVING
4 PEOPLE

INGREDIENTS

- **Medium bananas (2)**
- **Flaxseed meal (.25 cup)**
- **Nutmeg (1 tsp.)**
- **Peanut butter (.25 cup)**
- **Vanilla Greek yogurt (4 cups)**

DIRECTIONS

1. Peel and slice the bananas. Divide the yogurt into four serving dishes. Top each one with sliced bananas.
2. Microwave the peanut butter for 30 to 40 seconds until it's thoroughly melted. Drizzle the sauce over the banana slices and lightly dust them using the flaxseed meal and nutmeg to serve.

Nutritions: Calories: 370 Protein: 22.7 grams Fat: 10.6g

14. POACHED EGGS

PREPARATION AND COOKINGTIME
10 MINUTES

SERVING
2 PEOPLE

INGREDIENTS

- **Salt (.5 tsp.)**
- **Champagne vinegar (1 tsp.)**
- **Fresh eggs (2)**

DIRECTIONS

1. Prepare a cooking pot with cold water. Wait for it to boil using the medium temperature setting. Stir in the salt and vinegar.
2. Break each of the eggs into a ramekin. Place it close to the water and slide it out of the dish. Simmer until set.
3. Use a slotted spoon to lift it from the pan to help prevent sticking. Continue cooking until the yolk is runny and the white is cooked or about six minutes.
4. Prepare a container with ice water. Place the eggs into the bowl of ice water (It slows and stops the cooking process.)
5. Put them in paper towels to remove the water and serve.

Nutritions: *Calories: 72 Protein: 6.3 grams Fat: 5 grams*

15. PORTOBELLO PESTO EGG OMELETTE - GLUTEN-FREE

PREPARATION AND COOKINGTIME
25 MINUTES

SERVING
1 PEOPLE

INGREDIENTS

- **Olive oil (1 tsp.)**
- **Portobello mushroom cap (1)**
- **Red onion (.25 cup)**
- **Egg whites (4)**
- **Water (1 tsp.)**
- **Black pepper & salt (to taste)**
- **Prepared pesto (1 tsp.)**
- **Shredded low-fat mozzarella cheese (.25 cup)**

DIRECTIONS

1. Pour and warm the oil in a skillet using the medium temperature setting.
2. Chop and add the onions and mushrooms to sauté for about three to five minutes or until they're softened.
3. Crack the eggs into a bowl and whisk in the salt, pepper, and water. Dump the eggs on top of the onions and mushrooms.
4. Continue cooking for about five minutes, stirring occasionally. Sprinkle it using the cheese and top it off with some pesto.
5. Fold the omelet in half and continue cooking for about two to three more minutes before serving.

Nutritions: Calories: 259 Protein: 28 grams Fat: 12 grams

16. PROSCIUTTO - LETTUCE - TOMATO & AVOCADO SANDWICHES

PREPARATION AND COOKINGTIME
10-12 MINUTES

SERVING
4 PEOPLE

INGREDIENTS

- **Prosciutto (2 oz./8 thin slices)**
- **Ripe avocado (1 cut in half)**
- **Romaine lettuce (4 full leaves)**
- **Large ripe tomato (1)**
- **Whole grain or whole wheat bread slices (8)**
- **Black pepper and kosher salt (.25 tsp.)**

DIRECTIONS

1. Tear the lettuce leaves into eight pieces (total). Slice the tomato into eight rounds. Toast the bread and place it on a plate.
2. Scoop out the avocado flesh from the skin and toss it to a mixing bowl. Lightly dust it using the pepper and salt. Whisk or gently mash the avocado until it's creamy. Spread over the bread.
3. Make one sandwich. Take a slice of avocado toast; top it with a lettuce leaf, a prosciutto slice, and a tomato slice. Top with another slice of lettuce tomato and continue.
4. Repeat the process until all ingredients are depleted.

Nutritions: *Protein: 12 grams Fat: 9 grams Calories: 240*

17. PUMPKIN PANCAKES

PREPARATION AND COOKINGTIME
40 MINUTES

SERVING
6 PEOPLE

INGREDIENTS

- **Milk (1.5 cups)**
- **Egg (1)**
- **Vegetable oil (2 tbsp.)**
- **Pumpkin puree (1 cup)**
- **Vinegar (2 tbsp.)**
- **Baking soda (1 tsp.)**
- **Ground allspice (1 tsp.)**
- **All-purpose flour (2 cups)**
- **Brown sugar (3 tbsp.)**
- **Baking powder (2 tsp.)**
- **Salt (.5 tsp.)**
- **Ground ginger (.5 tsp.)**
- **Cinnamon (1 tsp.)**

DIRECTIONS

1. Whisk the egg, oil, vinegar, pumpkin, and the milk in a mixing bowl.
2. Mix the baking powder, salt, ginger, cinnamon, allspice, baking soda, brown sugar, and the flour in another container.
3. Stir the fixings in one bowl to combine.
4. Warm a frying pan or oiled griddle using the med-high heat setting.
5. Pour the batter into the griddle and brown. Serve them hot.

Nutritions: Calories: 278 Protein: 7.9 grams Fat: 7.2 grams

18. SCRAMBLED EGGS WITH ROASTED PEPPERS & GOAT CHEESE - GLUTEN-FREE

PREPARATION AND COOKINGTIME
15 MINUTES

SERVING
4 PEOPLE

INGREDIENTS

- **Olive oil (1.5 tsp.)**
- **Bell peppers (1 medium pepper / 1 cup)**
- **Garlic (2 cloves /1 tsp.)**
- **Large eggs (6)**
- **Sea salt (.25 tsp.)**
- **Water (2 tbsp.)**
- **Crumbled goat cheese (2 oz. / .5 cup)**
- **Chopped fresh mint (2 tbsp.)**

DIRECTIONS

1. Prepare a skillet using the med-high temperature setting on the stovetop. Add the oil. Once it's hot, toss in the peppers and sauté for five minutes.
2. Mince and stir in the garlic. Continue cooking for one minute.
3. Beat the water, eggs, and salt in a mixing container.
4. Reduce the temperature setting to med-low.
5. Empty the egg mixture over top of the peppers. Simmer it for one to two minutes until they're set on the bottom.
6. Sprinkle with the goat cheese and continue cooking for one to two more minutes. Stir until they are soft set.
7. Garnish with loosely packed fresh mint and serve.

Nutritions: *Calories: 201lt, Protein: 15 grams Fat: 15 grams*

19. SPINACH OMELET

PREPARATION AND COOKINGTIME
25-30 MINUTES

SERVING
4 PEOPLE

INGREDIENTS

- **Olive oil (3 tbsp.)**
- **Small onion (1)**
- **Garlic clove (1)**
- **Large tomatoes (4)**
- **Eggs (8)**
- **Black pepper (.25 tsp.)**
- **Fine sea salt (1 tsp.)**
- **Feta cheese (2 oz.**
- **Flat-leaf parsley (1 tbsp.)**

DIRECTIONS

1. Core and chop the tomatoes, parsley, and onion.
2. Set the oven to reach 400° Fahrenheit.
3. Pour the oil into an oven-proof skillet using the high heat temperature setting. Stir in the onions and sauté them until softened (5-7 min.).
4. Pour in the tomatoes, garlic, salt, and pepper.
5. Sauté the mixture for five more minutes and add the whisked eggs.
6. Stir and cook them for three to five minutes. When the bottom is set, put the skillet into the hot oven. Continue cooking for five additional minutes.
7. Transfer to the countertop and top it off with the parsley and feta. Serve the omelet warm.

Nutritions: Calories: 295 Protein: 15 grams Fat: 14 grams

20. YOGURT PARFAIT WITH ROASTED GRAPES & GREEK - GLUTEN-FREE

PREPARATION AND COOKINGTIME
30 MINUTES

SERVING
4 PEOPLE

INGREDIENTS

- **Seedless grapes (4 cups - 1.5 lbs.)**
- **Olive oil (1 tbsp.)**
- **2% Greek yogurt - plain (2**
- **ups)**
- **Honey (4 tsp.)**
- **Chopped walnuts (.5 cup)**

DIRECTIONS

1. Set the oven temperature to 450° Fahrenheit with the pan inside.
2. Rinse the grapes and discard the stems. Dab them using a towel and toss them with the oil.
3. Bake them for about 20 to 23 minutes until they are slightly shriveled. Stir about halfway through the cooking process.
4. Take the pan from the oven. Cool for five minutes.
5. Meanwhile, assemble the parfaits by adding the yogurt to the glass.
6. Once the grapes are cooled, garnish the yogurt using a teaspoon of honey, 2 tbsp. of the walnuts, and a portion of the grapes.
7. Prepare all four servings and serve or place in the fridge for later.

Nutritions: *Calories: 300 Protein: 7 grams Fat: 17 grams*

21. ZUCCHINI EGG WHITE FRITTATA

PREPARATION AND COOKINGTIME
25-30 MINUTES

SERVING
4 PEOPLE

INGREDIENTS

- **Olive oil (1 tsp.)**
- **Minced shallot (1 tbsp.)**
- **Minced garlic (1 clove)**
- **Zucchini (1 small)**
- **Egg whites (4)**
- **Black pepper and kosher salt (as desired)**
- **Freshly chopped thyme (.5tsp.)**

DIRECTIONS

1. Slice or shave the zucchini into strips. Chop the thyme.
2. Warm a skillet using the medium temperature setting and pour in the oil.
3. Mince and add the garlic and shallot to the skillet and sauté them for about five minutes. Stir in the zucchini. Continue cooking for about five minutes, stirring occasionally.
4. Whisk the salt, thyme, and egg whites together and mix into the zucchini mixture.
5. Continue cooking the mixture undisturbed for about two minutes using the low-temperature heat setting.
6. Flip the frittata and continue cooking one more minute.
7. Serve with a shake of salt and pepper to your desired taste.

Nutritions: Calories: 137 Protein: 16.5 grams Fat: 5 grams

2. MEDITERRANEAN LUNCHTIME & DINNER SALAD FAVORITES

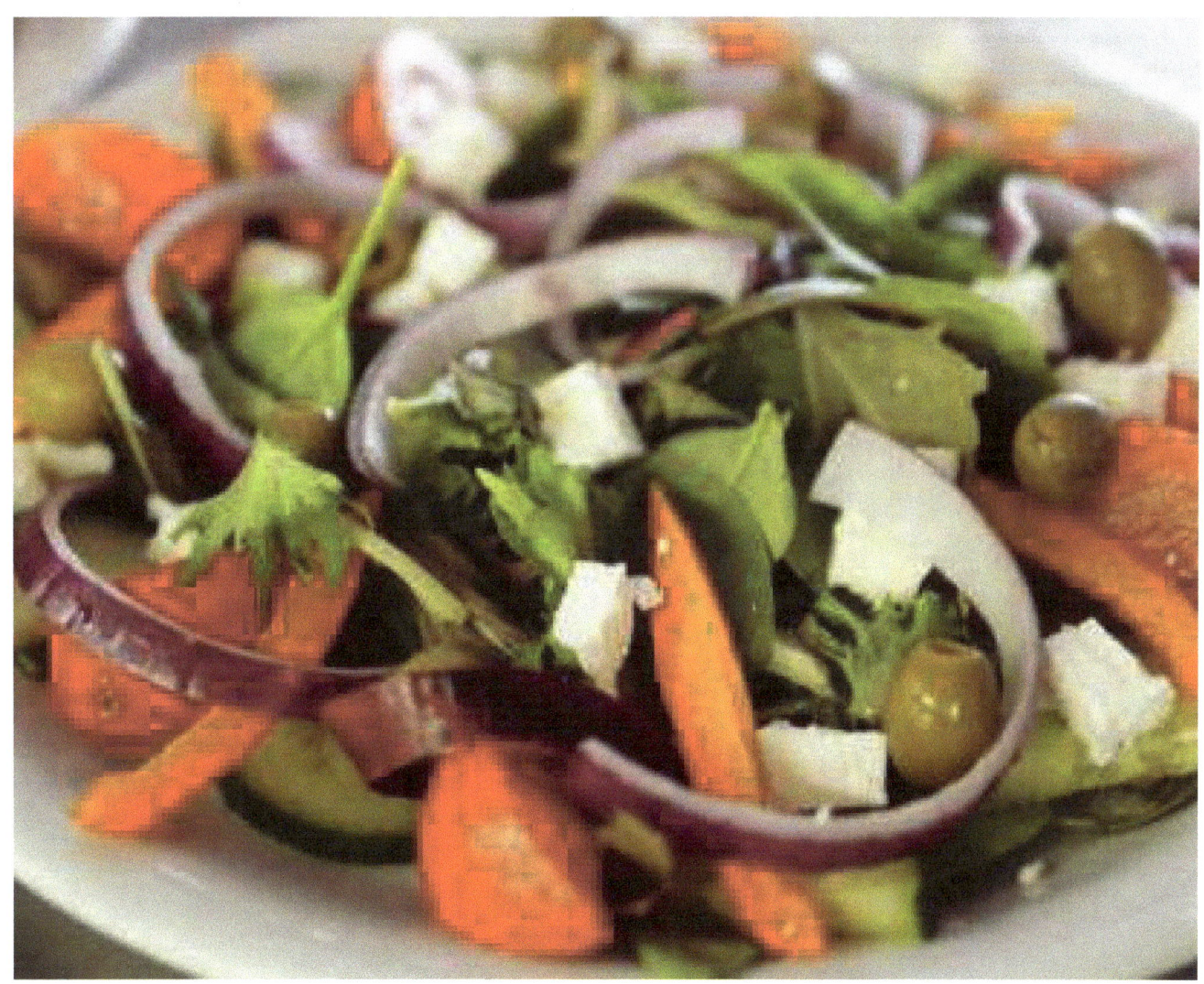

SALAD OPTIONS

1. ARUGULA SALAD

PREPARATION AND COOKINGTIME
15 MINUTES

SERVING
4 PEOPLE

INGREDIENTS

- **Arugula leaves (4 cups)**
- **Cherry tomatoes (1 cup)**
- **Pine nuts (.25 cup)**
- **Rice vinegar (1 tbsp.)**
- **Olive/Grapeseed oil (2 tbsp.)**
- **Salt & black pepper (as desired)**
- **Grated parmesan cheese (.25 cup)**
- **Large avocado (1 sliced)**

DIRECTIONS

1. Slice the avocado. Rinse and dry the arugula leaves.
2. Slice the cherry tomatoes into halves and grate the cheese.
3. Combine the arugula, tomatoes, pine nuts, and cheese into four salad containers.
4. Either place the slices to the side in another container or in a divided container for storage.
5. When it is time to serve, just add the oil and vinegar with a shake of pepper and salt.

Nutritions: Calories: 257 Protein: 6 grams Fat: 23 grams

2. ATHENIAN EGGPLANT SALAD

PREPARATION AND COOKINGTIME
1 HOUR 50 MIN

SERVING
8 PEOPLE

INGREDIENTS

- **Large eggplant (1)**
- **Olive oil (2 tbsp.)**
- **Tomato (1)**
- **Small onion (1)**
- **Distilled white vinegar (2 tbsp.)**
- **Fresh parsley (2 tbsp.)**
- **Feta cheese (.5 cup)**
- **Salt (as desired)**

DIRECTIONS

1. Preheat an outdoor grill using med-high heat.
2. Rinse and pierce the eggplant several times using a sharp knife or fork. Arrange it on the grill, turning often. The skin should be charred (15 min.). Set it aside to chill a few minutes.
3. Discard the seeds and chop the tomato. Dice/mince the onion and chop the parsley.
4. Remove the skin and dice the pulp from the eggplant. Toss it into a mixing bowl with the oil, vinegar, onion, tomato, parsley, and crumbled feta cheese, mixing thoroughly.
5. Pop it in the fridge for about an hour. Sprinkle using salt before serving.

Nutritions: *Fat: 6.9 grams Protein: 3.4 grams Calories: 99*

3. BARLEY SALAD

PREPARATION AND COOKINGTIME
1 HOUR 45 MIN

SERVING
6 PEOPLE

INGREDIENTS

- **Barley (1 cup)**
- **Water (2.5 cups)**
- **Olive oil (2 tbsp.)**
- **Garlic (2 cloves)**
- **Black olives (4 oz. can)**
- **Sun-dried tomatoes (7)**
- **Balsamic vinegar (1 tbsp.)**
- **Cilantro (.5 cup)**

DIRECTIONS

1. Pour the water and add the barley to cook using in a saucepan using the high-temperature setting.
2. Once it's boiling, lower the setting to med-low. Place a lid on the pot and simmer until the barley is tender (30 min.).
3. Drain the barley in a colander and cool to room temperature.
4. Puree the garlic, oil, tomatoes, and vinegar in a blender and add it to the barley.
5. Chop and mix in the olives and cilantro. Place a layer of foil or plastic over the container and refrigerate it to chill before serving.

Nutritions: Protein: 4.5 grams Fat: 11.8 grams Calories: 220

4. CHEESE TORTELLINI SALAD WITH SUN-DRIED TOMATOES

PREPARATION AND COOKINGTIME
42-45 MIN

SERVING
12 PEOPLE

INGREDIENTS

- **Cooked cheese tortellini (12 oz.)**
- **Halved grape tomatoes (2 cups)**
- **Kalamata olives (1 cup)**
- **Feta cheese (1 cubed cup)**
- **Diced red onion (.25 cup)**
- **Yellow/orange/red bell pepper (half of 1)**
- **Sun-dried tomatoes in oil & herbs (1 cup)**
- **Sicilian Lemon/white balsamic vinegar (.25 cup)**
- **Garlic olive oil (2 tbsp.)**
- **Zested lemon (1 medium)**
- **Olive oil (1.5 tbsp.)**
- **Basil leaves/chiffonade the leaves (12)**
- **Pepper and salt (as desired)**

DIRECTIONS

1. Cook the tortellini in salted boiling water, but don't overcook it.
2. Pour the tortellini in a large bowl and mix with the 1.5 tablespoons of olive oil and wait for it to cool.
3. Thinly slice the peppers and sun-dried tomatoes. Mix the sliced olives, halved grape tomatoes, pepper slivers, diced onion, sun-dried tomatoes, lemon zest, and feta cheese with the pasta.
4. Whisk the vinegar and garlic oil thoroughly and add it to the salad.
5. Toss and add the basil chiffonade. Taste test and serve.

Nutritions: *Calories: 205 Protein: 6 grams Fat: 12 grams*

5. CHICKPEA MEDITERRANEAN SALAD JARS

PREPARATION AND COOKINGTIME
15 MINUTES

SERVING
5 SMALL

INGREDIENTS

- **Olive oil (2 tbsp.)**
- **Lemon juice (.25 cup)**
- **Chickpeas (2 cans)**
- **Oil-packed julienned - sun-dried tomatoes - rinsed (.25 cup)**
- **Small red onion (1)**
- **Cherry tomatoes (.33 cup)**
- **Artichoke hearts (1 can)**
- **Finely chopped parsley (.33 cup)**
- **Dried thyme (1 tsp.)**

Optional:
- **Pepper (.5 tsp.)**
- **Salt (1 tsp.)**

DIRECTIONS

1. Drain and rinse the chickpeas and artichoke hearts. Slice/chop the onion and tomatoes.
2. Toss each of the fixings together and add the mixture into the chosen jars.
3. Place in the fridge for a quick snack for up to five days.

Nutritions: Calories: 224 Protein: 8 grams Fat: 10 grams

6. CUCUMBER SALAD

PREPARATION AND COOKINGTIME
5 MIN + CHILL TIME

SERVING
4 PEOPLE

INGREDIENTS

- **Cucumbers (5-6)**
- **Plain Greek yogurt (8 oz.)**
- **Garlic cloves (2)**
- **Oregano (1 tsp.)**
- **Fresh mint (1 tbsp.)**
- **Black pepper and Fine sea salt (.125 tsp. of each)**

DIRECTIONS

1. Slice the cucumbers. Mince the mint and garlic.
2. Mix the oregano, mint, garlic, yogurt, salt, and pepper with the cucumbers in a mixing bowl.
3. Place them in the fridge for approximately one hour before mealtime.

Nutritions: *Calories: 68 Protein: 1.45 grams Fat: 5.6 grams*

7. FETA - TOMATO SALAD

PREPARATION AND COOKINGTIME
20 MINUTES

SERVING
4 PEOPLE

INGREDIENTS

- **Balsamic vinegar (2 tbsp.)**
- **Freshly minced basil (1.5 tsp.) or Dried (.5 tsp.)**
- **Cherry or grape tomatoes (1 lb.)**
- **Crumbled feta cheese (.25 cup.)**
- **Coarsely chopped sweet onion (.5 cup)**
- **Salt (.5 tsp.)**
- **Olive oil (2 tbsp.)**

DIRECTIONS

1. Whisk the salt, basil, and vinegar.
2. Toss the onion into the vinegar mixture. Wait for about five minutes
3. Slice the tomatoes into halves and stir in the tomatoes, feta cheese, and oil type evenly. Serve.

Nutritions: Calories: 121 Protein: 3 grams Fat: 9 grams

8. GREEK FARRO SALAD

PREPARATION AND COOKINGTIME
1 HOUR

SERVING
6 PEOPLE

INGREDIENTS

The Salad:
- Pearled farro (1.5 cups)
- Water (1.25 cups)
- Olive oil (1 tbsp.)
- Low-sodium vegetable broth (2.5 cups)
- Baby spinach leaves (2 cups)
- Red onion (half of 1 small)
- Cucumber (1 medium - peeled)
- Green bell pepper (1 small)
- Cherry tomatoes (1 pint)
- Crumbled feta (.75 cup)
- Chickpeas (15 oz. can)

The Dressing:
- Honey (1 tbsp.)
- Fresh lemon juice (2 tbsp.)
- Vinegar - Red wine (1 tbsp.)
- Oregano (.25 tsp.)
- Red pepper flakes (1 pinch)
- Salt (.25 tsp.)
- Olive oil (.25 cup)

DIRECTIONS

1. Rinse and drain the chickpeas. Roughly chop the spinach. Squeeze the lemons for juice.
2. Prepare the Salad: Place a pot on the stovetop. Heat the oil over the medium temperature setting. Toss in the farro to cook for one minute, stirring often.
3. Pour in the broth and water. Once it's boiling, cover, place a lid on the pot, and lower the temperature setting to med-low. Simmer it for 30-35 minutes. Drain off any excess liquid and then transfer to a large mixing container.
4. Toss in the spinach and toss to wilt the spinach slightly. Wait for 15-20 minutes.
5. Slice the tomatoes into halves. Peel and thinly slice the cucumber, red onion, tomatoes, pepper, feta, and chickpeas. Toss everything well.
6. Whisk the dressing fixings until creamy smooth.
7. Pour some of the dressing into the bowl with the farro. Toss and add in more if desired.
8. Garnish and serve or chill for later.

Nutritions: *Protein: 13 grams Fat: 17 grams Calories: 365*

9. GREEK YOGURT CHICKEN SALAD STUFFED PEPPERS

PREPARATION AND COOKINGTIME
10-15 MINUTES

SERVING
6 PEOPLE

INGREDIENTS

- **Greek yogurt (.66 cup)**
- **Dijon mustard (2 tbsp.)**
- **Kosher salt & black pepper (as desired)**
- **Seasoned rice vinegar (2 tbsp.)**
- **Fresh parsley (.33 cup)**
- **Rotisserie chicken (1 cubed)**
- **Stalks of celery (4 sliced)**
- **Scallions - sliced and divided (1 bunch)**
- **Cherry tomatoes (1 pint - quartered & divided)**
- **English cucumber (half of 1 - diced)**
- **Bell peppers (3 halved with seeds removed)**

DIRECTIONS

1. Whisk the vinegar, salt, pepper, mustard, and yogurt in a mixing container. Chop and stir in the parsley.
2. Add the chicken, 3/4 of the scallions, celery, tomatoes, and cucumbers. Stir well.
3. Scoop out the bell pepper boats and divide the chicken salad into each one.
4. Garnish with the rest of the scallions, cucumbers, and tomatoes. Serve.

Nutritions: Calories: 116 Protein: 7 grams Fat: 3 grams

10. HERB ANTIPASTO PASTA SALAD PLATTER

PREPARATION AND COOKINGTIME
25 MINUTES

SERVING
8 PEOPLE

INGREDIENTS

- **Rainbow rotini (1 lb.)**
- **Grape tomatoes (1 pint)**
- **Crumbled feta cheese (8 oz.)**
- **Hard pepper salami (10 oz.)**
- **Kalamata olives (1 pint - ½ whole and ½ halved)**
- **Deli-sliced pepperoncini (8 oz.)**
- **Basil leaves (12 - cut into strips)**
- **Fresh oregano and rosemary (1 sprig each)**
- **Fresh thyme (5 sprigs)**
- **Greek Feta Salad dressing - ex Girand's (12 oz. bottle)**
- **Optional: Rosemary sprigs to garnish**

DIRECTIONS

1. Slice the tomatoes into halves and the salami into ⅛-inch slices (into strips). Slice half of the olives into halves. Chop the oregano and rosemary and remove the leaves from the thyme. Note: The pepperoncini is from a 16 oz. jar.
2. Prepare the pasta, leaving it under al dente. Add ¾ of the Greek dressing when it's cooled.
3. Toss in the tomatoes, salami, olives, 4 oz of feta, pepperoncini, and herbs.
4. Add in the rest of the dressing and wait for a few minutes for them to combine the flavors.
5. Scoop it out and top it off with the rest of the cheese. Decorate the plate with whole olives and garnishing of rosemary sprigs before serving.

Nutritions: *Calories: 543 Protein: 21 grams Fat: 28 grams*

11. HONEY LIME FRUIT SALAD

PREPARATION AND COOKINGTIME
5-7 MINUTES

SERVING
8 PEOPLE

INGREDIENTS

- **Sliced bananas (2 large)**
- **Fresh blueberries (.5 lb.)**
- **Fresh strawberries (1 lb.)**
- **Honey (2 tbsp.)**
- **Lime (1 juiced)**
- **Pine nuts (.33 cup)**

DIRECTIONS

1. Hull and slice the strawberries and bananas.
2. Combine the blueberries, strawberries, and bananas in a bowl.
3. Cross over it using the lime juice and honey.
4. Stir well and sprinkle with the nuts before serving.

Nutritions: Fat: 3.3 grams Protein: 2.4 grams Calories: 115

12. INSALATA CAPRESE II SALAD

PREPARATION AND COOKINGTIME
15 MINUTES

SERVING
6 PEOPLE

INGREDIENTS

- **Large ripened tomato (.25-inches thick - 4)**
- **Mozzarella cheese (.25-inches thick - 1 lb.)**
- **Fresh basil leaves (.33 cup)**
- **Olive oil (3 tbsp.)**
- **Black pepper & Fine sea salt (as desired)**

DIRECTIONS

1. Make the salad by layering and overlapping tomato slices with mozzarella cheese and leaves of basil.
2. Drizzle it with the oil, and a sprinkle of pepper and salt. Serve.

Nutritions: *Calories: 311 Protein: 17.9 grams Fat: 23.9 grams*

13. ITALIAN CELERY & ORANGE SALAD - GLUTEN-FREE

PREPARATION AND COOKINGTIME
15 MINUTES

SERVING
6 PEOPLE

INGREDIENTS

- **Celery stalks including the leaves (3)**
- **Large oranges (2)**
- **Green olives (.5 cup)**
- **Slice red onion (.25 cup)**
- **Olive oil (1 tbsp.)**
- **Brine from the olives (1 tbsp.)**
- **Fresh orange or lemon juice (1 tbsp.)**
- **Black pepper and Sea salt (.5 tsp.)**

DIRECTIONS

1. Slice the celery into .5-inch slices. Slice about .25 of one onion. Peel and slice the oranges into rounds. Squeeze the juice of choice.
2. Toss the onion, olives, oranges, and celery into a shallow bowl or large serving platter.
3. In another dish, whisk the lemon/orange juice, olive brine, and oil together.
4. Add the dressing, with a shake of pepper and salt before serving.

Nutritions: Fat: 4 grams Protein: 2 grams Calories: 65

14. MEDITERRANEAN PASTA SALAD

PREPARATION AND COOKINGTIME
25 MINUTES

SERVING
8 LARGE

INGREDIENTS

- Pasta - ex penne (12 oz.)
- Oil-packed sun-dried tomatoes (.5 cup)
- Marinated artichoke hearts (12-oz. jar)
- Kalamata olives (.5 cup)
- Capers (3 tbsp.)
- Scallions & fresh parsley (.25 cup of each)
- Packed - fresh arugula (1 cup)
- Parmesan cheese (.33 cup)
- Pine nuts (3 tbsp.)

The Dressing:
- Pesto - your choice (3 tbsp.)
- Olive oil (.33 cup)
- Reserved sun-dried tomato oil (2 tbsp.)
- Lemon juice (1 tbsp.)
- Black pepper & salt (as desired)

DIRECTIONS

1. Drain the tomatoes, reserving two tablespoons of the oil. Rinse the capers. Chop the olives, scallions, and parsley. Drain and chop the artichokes. Prepare the pasta according to package directions until it's al dente. Rinse and drain the pasta and wait for it to cool.
2. Combine and toss the olives, artichoke hearts, pasta, sun-dried tomatoes, scallions, capers, and parsley.
3. In a small mixing container, combine the oil, pesto, juice, sun-dried tomato oil, pepper, and salt. Stir thoroughly and wait for it to chill in the refrigerator until serving time.
4. Time to Eat: Add the arugula, pine nuts, and parmesan into the salad and toss to combine. Serve with the dressing.

Nutritions: Calories: 259 Protein: 6.7 grams Fat: 20 grams

15. SALAD IN A SANDWICH

PREPARATION AND COOKINGTIME
20 MINUTES

SERVING
4 PEOPLE

INGREDIENTS

- **Small tomatoes (12 oz.)**
- **Small spinach leaves (6 cups)**
- **English hothouse cucumber (1.5 cups)**
- **Feta cheese (1 cup - crumbled)**
- **Kalamata olives - pitted black brine-cured (.33 cup)**
- **Basil (16 leaves)**
- **Olive oil (.25 cup)**
- **Fresh lemon juice (5 tsp.)**
- **Garlic clove (1 large)**
- **Pita bread rounds (4 toasted)**

DIRECTIONS

1. Thinly slice the tomatoes and place them in a colander to drain for 15 minutes. Thinly slice the cucumber and basil leaves. Coarsely chop the olives and mince the clove of garlic. Trim the stems from the spinach.
2. Combine the spinach, olives, tomatoes, cucumber, feta cheese, and basil in a large mixing container.
3. Whisk oil, salt, pepper, juice, and garlic in another dish to blend.
4. Spritz the salad using the dressing and toss it thoroughly to cover.
5. Cut the pita bread rounds in half (crosswise).
6. Load the salad into the pita halves. Serve with a smile!

Nutritions: Calories: 462 Protein: 16.3 grams Fat: 22 grams

16. SHRIMP ORZO SALAD - MEDITERRANEAN -STYLE

PREPARATION AND COOKINGTIME
30 MINUTES

SERVING
8 PEOPLE

INGREDIENTS

- **Cooked shrimp (.75 lb.)**
- **Orzo pasta (16 oz. pkg.)**
- **Red onion (.75 cup)**
- **Green pepper (1 cup)**
- **Water-packed artichoke hearts (14 oz. can)**
- **Sweet red pepper (1 cup)**
- **Freshly minced parsley (.5 cup)**
- **Pitted Greek olives (.5 cup)**
- **Freshly chopped dill (.33 cup)**
- **Greek vinaigrette (.75 cup)**

DIRECTIONS

1. Peel, devein, and cook the shrimp. Slice each one into thirds (31-40-count). Finely chop the onions and peppers.
2. Prepare the orzo using the manufacturer's directions. Rinse and drain the orzo with cold water.
3. Combine the shrimp, orzo, olives, herbs, and veggies.
4. Sprinkle with vinaigrette and toss to coat.
5. Refrigerate and cover. Serve as a delicious side salad or for lunch.

Nutritions: Calories: 397 Protein: 18 grams Fat: 12 grams

17. 3-INGREDIENT MEDITERRANEAN SALAD

PREPARATION AND COOKINGTIME
10 MINUTES

SERVING
4 PEOPLE

INGREDIENTS

- **Diced - Roma tomatoes (6 or about 3 cups)**
- **Large English or hot-house cucumber (1 large - diced)**
- **Freshly chopped parsley leaves (.5 to .75 packed cup)**
- **Salt (as desired)**
- **Black pepper (.5 tsp.)**
- **Olive oil (2 tbsp.)**
- **Ground sumac (1 tsp.)**
- **Lemon juice (2 tsp.)**

DIRECTIONS

1. Dice the tomatoes and cucumbers. Mix them with the parsley in a large salad container.
2. Dust the salad using salt and set it to the side for about four minutes.
3. Toss all of the fixings and toss them with the salad.
4. Wait a few minutes and serve it.

Nutritions: Protein: 2.3 grams Fat: 7.5 grams Calories: 105

18. TOMATO SALAD - GRILLED HALLOUMI & HERBS

PREPARATION AND COOKINGTIME
15 MINUTES

SERVING
4 PEOPLE

INGREDIENTS

- **Tomatoes - sliced into rounds (1 lb.)**
- **Lemon (half of 1)**
- **Black pepper & Flaky salt (as desired)**
- **Olive oil (as desired)**
- **Halloumi cheese (.5 lb. - sliced into 4 slabs)**
- **Basil leaves (5 torn)**
- **Flat-leaf parsley (2 tbsp.)**

DIRECTIONS

1. Heat a grill pan using the medium-high temperature setting.
2. Place some tomatoes on a serving platter in the serving dishes. Lightly squeeze with the lemon and season with the pepper and salt.
3. Brush the grill with the oil and add the cheese. Prepare and flip it once during the process (1 minute). Add it to the top of the tomatoes.
4. Spritz using oil and sprinkle of finely chopped parsley and basil. Serve it immediately.

Nutritions: Calories: 196 Protein: 9 grams Fat: 15 grams

19. TUNA ANTIPASTO SALAD

PREPARATION AND COOKINGTIME
25 MINUTES

SERVING
4 PEOPLE

INGREDIENTS

- **Beans - ex. black-eyed peas/ chickpeas/kidney beans, rinsed (1 15- to 19-oz. can)**
- **Chunk light tuna - Water-packed (2 - 5-6-oz. cans)**
- **Red bell pepper (1 large)**
- **Red onion (.5 cup)**
- **Fresh parsley - divided (.5 cup)**
- **Capers (4 tsp.)**
- **Fresh rosemary (1.5 tsp.)**
- **Lemon juice, divided (.5 cup)**
- **Olive oil - divided (4 tbsp.)**
- **Freshly ground pepper (as desired)**
- **Salt (.25 tsp.)**
- **Mixed salad greens (8 cups)**

DIRECTIONS

1. Rinse the beans, capers, and greens. Drain and flake the tuna.
2. Finely chop the bell pepper, onion, parsley, and rosemary.
3. Combine the tuna, ¼ cup lemon juice, onion, bell pepper, capers, pepper, salt, parsley, rosemary, beans, and two tablespoons of oil in a mixing container.
4. Whisk the remaining two tablespoons of oil and ¼ cup of the juice in a large mixing container. Toss in the greens and churn to mix.
5. Divide the greens into the salad dishes and add the salad.

Nutritions: Calories: 306 Protein: 14.8 grams Fat: 15.9 grams

20. TURKISH ORANGE SALAD WITH MEDITERRANEAN DRESSING

PREPARATION AND COOKINGTIME
20 MINUTES

SERVING
4 PEOPLE

INGREDIENTS

- **Oranges (4)**
- **Blood oranges (3)**
- **Onion (1 small)**
- **Lemon juice (2 tbsp.)**
- **Olive oil (3 tbsp.)**
- **Salt (as desired)**
- **Freshly cracked black pepper (1 pinch)**
- **Dried black olives (10)**

DIRECTIONS

1. Slice a little piece off the top and bottom of each orange to create an even cutting surface. Remove all skin and pith without taking too much off the fruit.
2. Horizontally slice oranges and arrange on a serving platter.
3. Finely dice the onion and combine the juice, salt, and oil in a mixing bowl. Dump the mixture over the oranges. Grind fresh pepper over the salad and arrange black olives on top to serve.

Nutritions: Calories: 186 Protein: 1.8 grams Fat: 11.7 grams

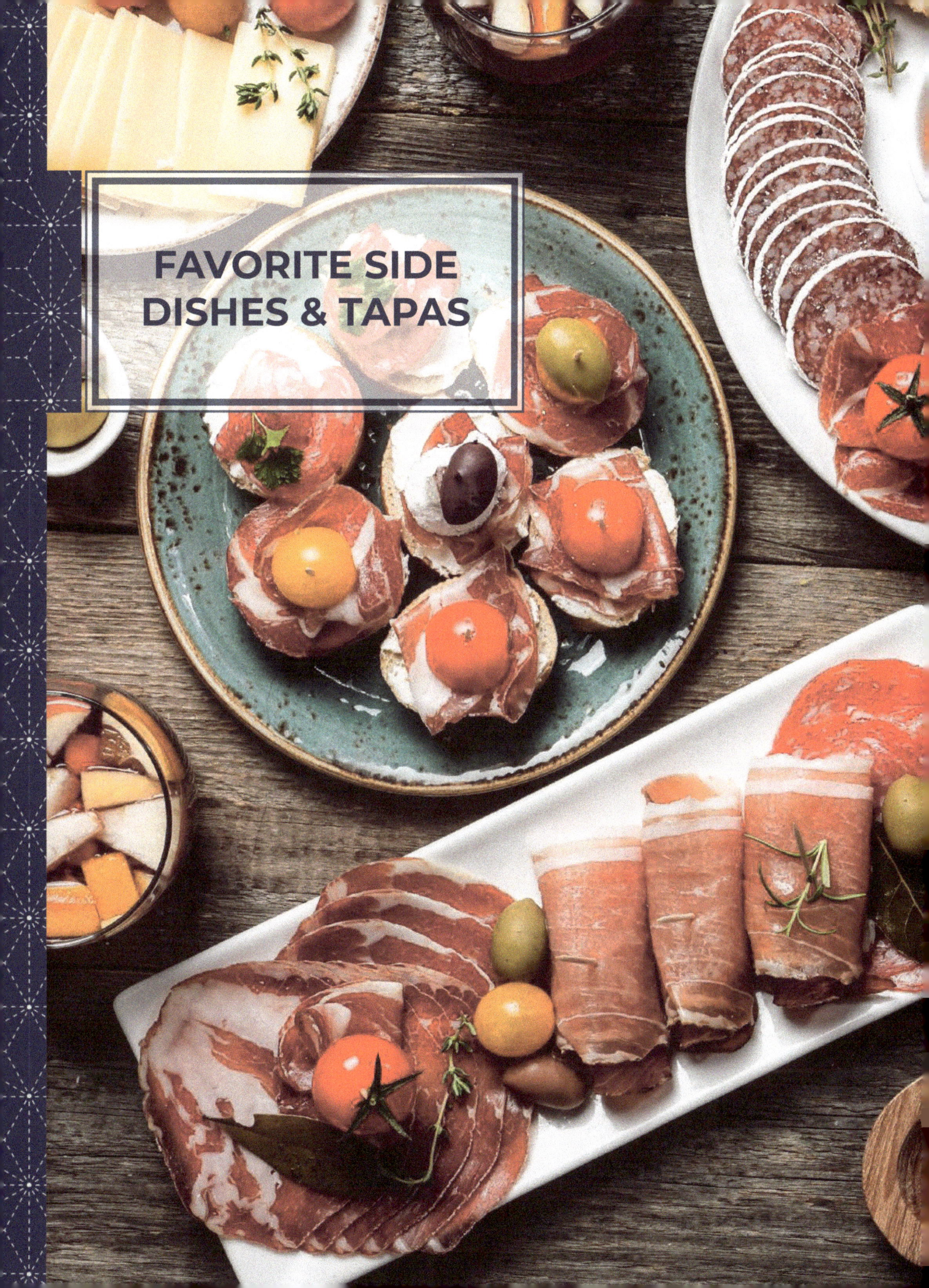

FAVORITE SIDE DISHES & TAPAS

1. AVOCADO & TUNA TAPAS

PREPARATION AND COOKINGTIME
10 MINUTES

SERVING
4 PEOPLE

INGREDIENTS

- **Solid white tuna packed in water (12 oz. can)**
- **Green onions (3 + more for garnish)**
- **Red bell pepper (half of 1)**
- **Garlic salt and black pepper (as desired)**
- **Mayonnaise (1 tbsp.)**
- **Balsamic vinegar (1 dash)**
- **Ripe avocados (2)**

DIRECTIONS

1. Drain the tuna thoroughly. Remove the pit and slice the avocados into halves.
2. Chop the bell pepper, and thinly slice the onions. Whisk the vinegar, red pepper, onions, salt, pepper, mayonnaise, and tuna.
3. Load the avocado halves with the tuna.
4. Top it off with a portion of green onions and black pepper before serving.

Nutritions: Calories: 194 Protein: 23.9 grams Fat: 18.2 grams

2. CANNELLINI BEAN LETTUCE WRAPS

PREPARATION AND COOKINGTIME
15 MINUTES

SERVING
4 PEOPLE

INGREDIENTS

- **Olive oil (1 tbsp.)**
- **Red onion (.5 cup)**
- **Tomatoes (1 medium/.75 cup)**
- **Freshly cracked black pepper (.25 tsp.)**
- **Fresh curly parsley (.25 cup)**
- **Great Northern beans or cannellini beans (15 oz. can)**
- **Prepared hummus (.5 cup)**
- **Romaine lettuce leaves (8)**

DIRECTIONS

1. Drain and rinse the vegetables and beans. Chop the tomatoes and onion into fine pieces.
2. Add the oil into a skillet to heat using the medium heat temperature setting.
3. Chop and toss in the onions, tomatoes, and pepper to sauté for six. Stir occasionally.
4. Pour in the drained beans and simmer them for three additional minutes.
5. Mix in the parsley after removing it from the burner.
6. Spread the hummus over each of the leaves of lettuce. Spread the bean mixture to the center of each leaf. Fold it over to make a wrap to serve.

Nutritions: Calories: 235 Protein: 4 grams Fat: 20 grams

3. EASY FARFALLE WITH FRESH TOMATOES

PREPARATION AND COOKINGTIME
25-30 MINUTES

SERVING
4 PEOPLE

INGREDIENTS

- **Tomatoes (4/2 lb. total weight)**
- **Fresh basil (.5 cup)**
- **Red onion (3 tbsp.)**
- **Garlic (1 clove)**
- **Olive oil (3 tbsp.)**
- **Red wine vinegar (1 tbsp.)**
- **Black pepper (.25 tsp.)**
- **Salt (.75 tsp.)**
- **Farfalle pasta (.5 lb.)**

DIRECTIONS

1. Peel and remove the seeds from the tomatoes and dice them into ½-inch pieces. Cut the basil into slender ribbons, using the whole leaves for garnishing. Chop/mince the garlic and onion.
2. Prepare the sauce in a large mixing container using the tomatoes, onion, basil oil, garlic, vinegar, pepper, and salt. Toss to mix.
3. Prepare a large pot of water (about ¾ full) and wait for it to boil. Toss in the farfalle and simmer until it's al dente (10 min.) Pour it into a colander to drain.
4. Divide the pasta and sauce between the bowls and serve.

Nutritions: Calories: 212.5 Protein: 4.2 grams Fat: 11.2 grams

4. FRIED RICE WITH SPINACH - PEPPERS & ARTICHOKES

PREPARATION AND COOKINGTIME
15-20 MINUTES

SERVING
4 PEOPLE

INGREDIENTS

- **Cooked rice (1.5 cups)**
- **Frozen chopped spinach (10 oz.)**
- **Marinated artichoke hearts (6 oz.)**
- **Roasted red peppers (4 oz.)**
- **Minced garlic (.5 tsp.)**
- **Crumbled feta cheese with herbs (.5 cup)**
- **Olive oil (2 tbsp.)**

DIRECTIONS

1. Prepare the vegetables. Mince the garlic. Thaw and drain the frozen spinach. Drain and quarter the artichoke hearts. Drain and chop the roasted red peppers.
2. Heat a skillet on the stovetop to warm the oil using the medium heat setting. Toss in the garlic to sauté for two minutes.
3. Toss in the rice and continue cooking for about two minutes until well heated.
4. Fold in the spinach and continue cooking for three more minutes.
5. Add the red peppers and artichoke hearts. Simmer for two minutes.
6. Stir in the feta cheese and serve immediately.

Nutritions: Calories: 244 Protein: 9.3 grams Fat: 12.9 grams

5. GIGANTES (GREEK LIMA BEANS)

PREPARATION AND COOKINGTIME
10 HOURS

SERVING
8 PEOPLE

INGREDIENTS

- **Also Needed: 9 x 13 baking dish**
- **Dried lima beans (16 oz. pkg.)**
- **Chopped tomatoes with juice (2 - 16 oz. cans)**
- **Olive oil (1 cup)**
- **Minced garlic (3 cloves)**
- **Sea salt (as desired)**
- **Freshly chopped dill (1 tsp.)**

DIRECTIONS

1. Pour the beans into a large saucepan with water to fill two inches over the top of the beans. Set them aside to soak overnight.
2. Set the oven at 375° Fahrenheit.
3. Place the saucepan over medium heat and wait for it to boil. Once it's boiling, lower the temperature setting to med-low and simmer for 20 minutes. Dump the water and drain the beans in a colander.
4. Pour and fold the beans into the baking dish with the dill, salt, oil, garlic, and tomatoes.
5. Bake the beans for 1.5 to 2 hours. Add water as needed, stirring occasionally.

Nutritions: Calories: 449 Protein: 13 grams Fat: 27.5 grams

6. GLUTEN-FREE SPANISH RICE

PREPARATION AND COOKINGTIME
40 MINUTES

SERVING
6 PEOPLE

INGREDIENTS

- **Olive oil (1 tbsp.)**
- **Garlic (2 cloves)**
- **Medium onion (.5 cup)**
- **Medium green bell pepper (.5 cup)**
- **Long-grain rice - regular/ uncooked (1 cup)**
- **Sea salt (.25 tsp.)**
- **Crushed red pepper (.25 tsp.)**
- **Chicken broth (1.75 cups)**
- **Undrained - Diced fire-roasted tomatoes (1 - 14.5 oz. can)**
- **Also Needed: 3-quart saucepan**

DIRECTIONS

1. Heat the oil in the saucepan using the medium temperature setting.
2. Chop/dice the onion, garlic, and bell pepper and toss them into the skillet for about five minutes, stirring constantly.
3. Add in the red pepper, salt, broth (reduced-sodium is best), rice, and tomatoes. Wait for it to boil. Reduce the temperature setting and cook until the rice is tender before serving (20-25 min.).

Nutritions: Calories: 170 Protein: 4 grams Fat: 2.5 grams

7. GREEK BAKED ZUCCHINI & POTATOES - BRIAM

PREPARATION AND COOKINGTIME
2 HOURS

SERVING
4 PEOPLE

INGREDIENTS

- **Potatoes (2 lb.)**
- **Zucchini (4 large)**
- **Red onions (4 small)**
- **Ripe tomatoes (6 pureed)**
- **Olive oil (.5 cup)**
- **Optional: Freshly chopped parsley (2 tbsp.)**
- **Black pepper & Sea salt (to taste)**
- **Also Needed: 9 by 13-inch or larger baking dish**

DIRECTIONS

1. Thinly slice the zucchini, onions, and potatoes.
2. Set the oven to reach 400° Fahrenheit.
3. Chop and spread the red onions, zucchini, and potatoes in the baking pan.
4. Cover with pureed tomatoes, parsley, and olive oil.
5. Sprinkle using the salt and pepper. Toss until evenly coated.
6. Bake them for approximately one hour or until the veggies are moist and softened.
7. Cool them slightly and serve at room temperature.

Nutritions: Calories: 534 Protein: 11.3 grams Fat: 28.3 grams

8. GREEN BEANS & FETA

PREPARATION AND COOKINGTIME
15 MINUTES

SERVING
8 PEOPLE

INGREDIENTS

- **Olive oil (2 tbsp.)**
- **Freshly trimmed green beans (1 lb.)**
- **Red onion (2 tbsp.)**
- **Tarragon vinegar (1 tbsp.)**
- **Salt (.5 tsp.)**
- **Pepper (.25 tsp.)**
- **Garlic (1 clove)**
- **Crumbled feta cheese (.5 cup or 2 oz.)**
- **Also Needed: 6-quart saucepan**

DIRECTIONS

1. Add one inch of water into the pan and add the beans.
2. Finely chop the onion and garlic and add the rest of the fixings (omit the cheese) to simmer for eight to ten minutes with the lid off. Drain.
3. Scoop the beans into a serving dish and add the cheese.
4. Toss and serve warm.

Nutritions: Fat: 5 grams Protein: 2 grams Calories: 80

9. KALE - MEDITERRANEAN-STYLE

PREPARATION AND COOKINGTIME
15 MINUTES

SERVING
6 PEOPLE

INGREDIENTS

- **Chopped kale (12 cups)**
- **Olive oil (1 tbsp./as needed)**
- **Minced garlic (1 tbsp.)**
- **Salt and black pepper (as preferred)**
- **Soy sauce (1 tsp.)**
- **Lemon juice (2 tbsp.)**

DIRECTIONS

1. Prepare a saucepan with a steamer insert. Pour in plenty of water to cover the bottom.
2. Put a lid on the pot and boil using the high-temperature setting.
3. Toss in the kale. Once it boils, time for 7-10 minutes. Drain.
4. Whisk the soy sauce, lemon juice, garlic, oil, black pepper, and salt. Toss in the steamed kale. Toss until coated and serve.

Nutritions: Calories: 91 Protein: 4.6 grams Fat: 3.2 grams

10. MEDITERRANEAN ENDIVE BOATS

PREPARATION AND COOKINGTIME
10 MINUTES

SERVING
8 PEOPLE

INGREDIENTS

- **Chopped sun-dried tomatoes (.33 cup)**
- **Chickpeas (.66 cup)**
- **Olive oil (1 tbsp.)**
- **Crumbled feta (.25 cup)**
- **Chopped basil leaves (3)**
- **Balsamic reduction (2 tbsp.)**

DIRECTIONS

1. Rinse and drain the chickpeas.
2. Combine the oil, with the drained chickpeas, and tomatoes.
3. Cut the base of the endive and pull the leaves apart. (It should make eight.)
4. Arrange the leaves on the serving platter and add the chickpea mixture.
5. Garnish it with the crumbled feta, and top it off with chopped basil and a spritz of balsamic reduction.

Nutritions: Calories: 715 Protein: 32 grams Fat: 30 gram

11. MEDITERRANEAN NACHOS

PREPARATION AND COOKINGTIME
10 MINUTES

SERVING
6 PEOPLE

INGREDIENTS

- **Kalamata olives (2 tbsp.)**
- **Sun-dried tomatoes in oil (2 tbsp. + 2 tsp. oil)**
- **Drained Roma- small plum tomato (1 medium)**
- **Green onion (1 tbsp.)**
- **Tortilla chips (4 oz./30 chips approx.)**
- **Feta cheese (4 oz.)**

DIRECTIONS

1. Prep the fixings. Thinly slice/chop the onion olives, and tomatoes. Mix the sun-dried tomatoes, olives, oil, onions, and plum tomato. Set them aside for now.
2. Place the tortillas (single-layered) on a microwavable platter. Crumble the feta over the chips.
3. Cook in the microwave for one minute on high.
4. Rotate the dish and continue cooking for another 30 to 60 seconds or until it's bubbly.
5. Spoon the tomato mixture over the chips and serve.

Nutritions: Calories: 170 Protein: 4 grams Fat: 11 grams

12. MEDITERRANEAN POTATOES

PREPARATION AND COOKING TIME
45-50 MINUTES

SERVING
4 PEOPLE

INGREDIENTS

- **Medium potatoes (4-5)**
- **Olive oil (1 tbsp.)**
- **Butter (1 tbsp. - melted)**
- **Greek seasoning (6 tsp.)**
- **Garlic seasoning (.125 tsp.)**
- **Also Needed: 9 x 13-inch casserole dish**

DIRECTIONS

1. Set the oven temperature to 350° Fahrenheit.
2. Cube the potatoes and toss them into the dish with the rest of the fixings.
3. Bake them for 30-40 minutes. Turn occasionally.
4. Serve when the potatoes are browned to your liking.

Nutritions: Calories: 207.8 Protein: 3.8 grams Fat: 6.3 grams

13. MELITZANES IMAM/GREEK EGGPLANT DISH

PREPARATION AND COOKINGTIME
1 HOUR 15 MIN

SERVING
2 PEOPLE

INGREDIENTS

- **Eggplant (1)**
- **Diced tomatoes, drained (14.5 oz. can)**
- **Tomato paste (1 tbsp.)**
- **Medium onion (1)**
- **Minced garlic (1 tbsp./to taste)**
- **Ground cinnamon (1 tsp.)**
- **Pepper & salt (as desired)**
- **Olive oil (3 tbsp.)**

DIRECTIONS

1. Set the oven to reach 350° Fahrenheit.
2. Slice the eggplant - lengthwise - in half. Cut out the halves leaving about a one-inch shell. Set the flesh aside.
3. Arrange the shells on a baking pan. Lightly spritz the eggplant using oil and bake until softened (30 min.).
4. Chop the leftover eggplant into small pieces.
5. Prepare a skillet using the medium temperature setting with two tablespoons of oil.
6. Dice and add the onion, garlic, and chopped eggplant to sauté for a few minutes.
7. Dump the tomato paste and tomatoes and simmer using the low-heat temperature setting.
8. Transfer the shells to the countertop, and spoon in the tomato/eggplant mixture. Sprinkle using cinnamon and bake for another 30 minutes and serve.

Nutritions: Calories: 314 Protein: 5.3 grams Fat: 20.8 grams

14. RED MEDITERRANEAN POTATO SALAD

PREPARATION AND COOKINGTIME
25 MINUTES

SERVING
12 PEOPLE

INGREDIENTS

- **Red potatoes (1.5 lb. - halved)**
- **Bacon (3 slices)**
- **Grape tomatoes - red/yellow (.75 cup)**
- **Chopped onion (.25 cup)**
- **Sliced olives (.25 cup)**
- **Fat-free Italian dressing (.5 cup)**
- **Cider vinegar (1 tbsp.)**
- **Italian parsley (1 tbsp.)**
- **Also Needed: 3-quart saucepan**

DIRECTIONS

1. Pour about one inch of water into the pan and let it boil.
2. Slice and toss in the potatoes. Place a lid on the pot and cook them using the medium temperature setting for 10-15 minutes until tender. Drain and slightly cool.
3. Slice the halved potatoes into .75-inch cubes and toss them into a salad dish.
4. Prepare a microwave-safe platter with a layer of paper towels. Add in the bacon and cook on high for two to three minutes. Crumble them.
5. Stir the tomatoes, bacon, onion, and olives in with the potatoes.
6. Whisk the vinegar and dressing. Pour over the potatoes and gently toss.
7. Chop the parsley to sprinkle the salad, and serve or chill.

Nutritions: Fat: 1.5 grams Protein: 2 grams Calories: 60

15. SAVORY MEDITERRANEAN ORZO

PREPARATION AND COOKINGTIME
45 MINUTES

SERVING
12-3/4 CUP PORTION

INGREDIENTS

- **Chicken broth - reduced sodium (4 cups)**
- **Orzo pasta (16 oz. pkg.)**
- **Medium onion (1)**
- **Olive oil (2 tbsp.)**
- **Garlic (4 cloves)**
- **Crumbled feta cheese - divided (8 oz./2 cups)**
- **Roasted sweet red peppers (7.5 oz. jar)**
- **Frozen - chopped spinach (10 oz. pkg.)**
- **Yellow summer squash (1 small - finely chopped)**
- **Salt and black pepper (.5 tsp. each)**
- **Also Needed: 13 by 9-inch baking dish**

DIRECTIONS

1. Grease the baking dish and set it to the side for now.
2. Pour water into a large saucepan and wait for it to boil. Stir in orzo; cook over medium heat until tender (six to eight minutes). Place the pan on the countertop, off of the burner.
3. Prepare a pan with oil. Dice and sauté the onion until tender. Mince and add the garlic, sautéing it for one minute longer.
4. Drain and chop the jarred peppers. Thaw and squeeze the spinach to remove the liquids. Stir one cup of cheese, squash, red peppers, spinach, salt, and pepper into the orzo mixture.
5. Dump the mixture into the baking dish, sprinkling it with the rest of the cheese. Bake it without the lid, at 350° Fahrenheit for 20 to 25 minutes until it's thoroughly heated.

Nutritions: Fat: 6 grams Protein: 10 grams Calories: 233

16. SPINACH PIE

PREPARATION AND COOKINGTIME
60 MINUTES

SERVING
6 PEOPLE

INGREDIENTS

- **Melted butter (.5 cup)**
- **Frozen spinach (10 oz. pkg.)**
- **Fresh parsley (.5 cup)**
- **Green onions (.5 cup)**
- **Fresh dill (.5 cup)**
- **Crumbled feta cheese (.5 cup)**
- **Cream cheese (4 oz.)**
- **Cottage cheese (4 oz.)**
- **Parmesan (2 tbsp. - grated)**
- **Large eggs (2)**
- **Pepper and salt (as desired)**
- **Phyllo dough (40 sheets)**

DIRECTIONS

1. Heat the oven setting at 350° Fahrenheit.
2. Mince/chop the onions, dill, and parsley. Thaw the spinach and sheets of dough. Dab the spinach dry by squeezing.
3. Combine the spinach, scallions, eggs, cheeses, parsley, dill, pepper, and salt in a blender until it's creamy.
4. Prepare the small phyllo triangles by filling them with one teaspoon of the spinach mixture.
5. Lightly brush the outside of the triangles with butter and arrange them with the seam-side facing downwards on an ungreased baking tray.
6. Place them in the heated oven to bake until golden brown and puffed (20-25 min.). Serve piping hot.

Nutritions: Calories: 555 Protein: 18.7 grams Fat: 21.3 grams

3. MEDITERRANEAN LUNCHTIME & DINNER SOUP FAVORITES

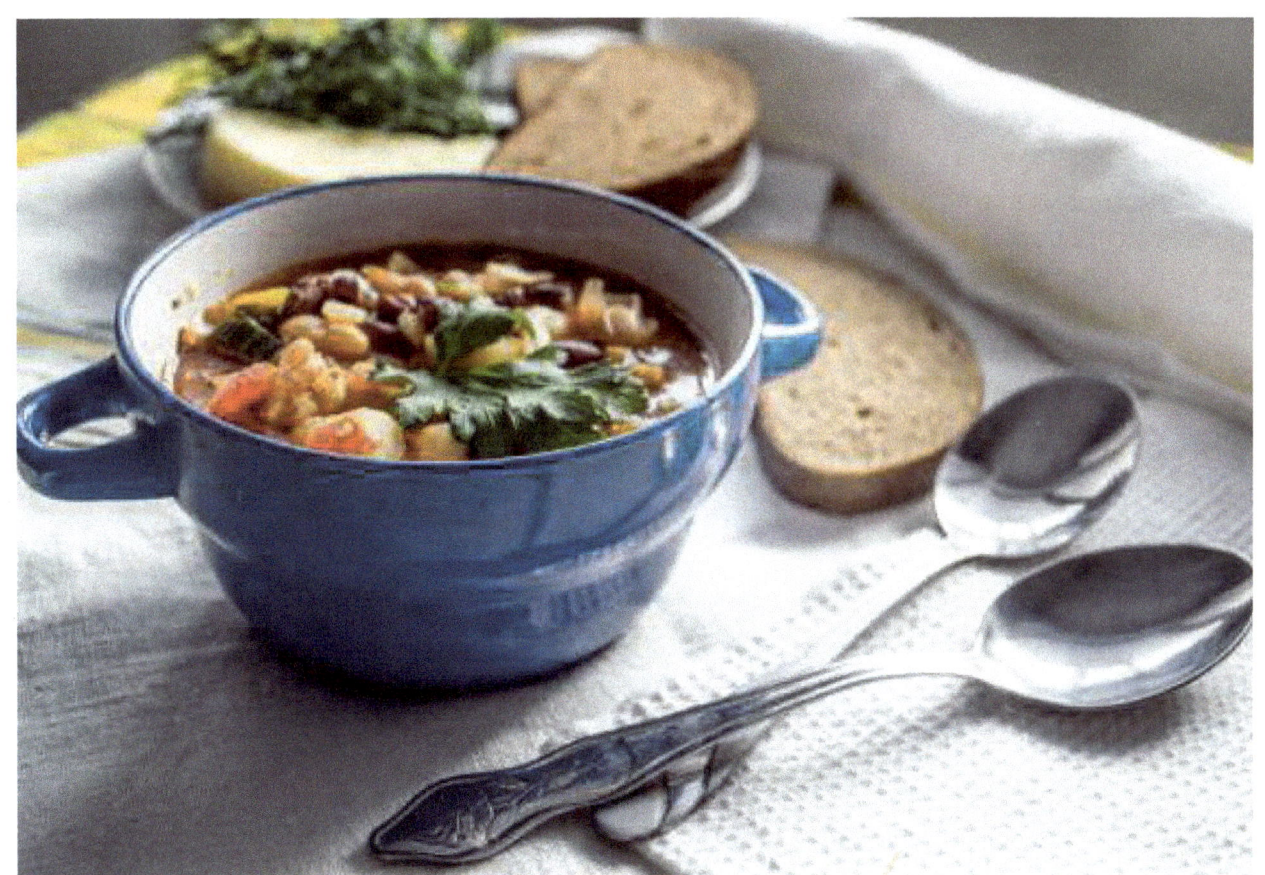

1. AJOBLANCO (COLD SPANISH ALMOND SOUP)

PREPARATION AND COOKINGTIME
25 MINUTES

SERVING
4 PEOPLE

INGREDIENTS

- **Blanched almonds (1 lb.)**
- **Red wine vinegar (3 tbsp.)**
- **Olive oil (6 tbsp.)**
- **Ice-cold water (3 tbsp.)**
- **Garlic (1 clove)**
- **Salt (as desired)**
- **Green grapes (.25 cup)**

DIRECTIONS

1. Mince the garlic and peel the grapes.
2. Combine the oil, almonds, vinegar, water, salt, and garlic in a blender until it's creamy, adding water as needed to keep it thick, but pourable.
3. Wait for about 15 minutes and chill the delicious soup before garnishing with the grapes.

Nutritions: Calories: 853 Protein: 25 grams Fat: 77.8 grams

2. CHICKPEA - HARISSA STEW & EGGPLANT WITH MILLET

PREPARATION AND COOKINGTIME
60-70 MINUTES

SERVING
2 PEOPLE

INGREDIENTS

- **Kosher salt (1 pinch)**
- **Water (2 cups)**
- **Freshly cracked black pepper (as desired)**
- **Millet (1 cup)**
- **Ghee/neutral high-heat oil - divided (2 tbsp.)**
- **Large Japanese eggplant (1)**
- **Garlic cloves (3)**
- **Onion (1)**
- **Pureed tomatoes (14 oz. can)**
- **Chickpeas - drained (14 oz. can)**
- **Harissa paste (2 tbsp.)**
- **For the Garnish: Cilantro (1 bunch)**

DIRECTIONS

1. Pour the water, salt, and millet into a saucepan. Wait for it to boil and place a lid on the pot to cook for about 25 minutes. When done, gently fluff with a fork and let it cool.
2. While that is cooling, pour in one tablespoon of oil or ghee in a deep skillet using the medium heat setting. Toss in the eggplant, salt, and pepper.
3. Cook it until tender and golden brown, adding more ghee as needed (10 min.). Dump the eggplant into a container and set it to the side for now.
4. Add the rest of the ghee into the same pan. Mince and toss in the onion to sauté for about 8 to 10 minutes.
5. Mince and stir in the garlic and simmer for another two minutes. Pour in the chickpeas, tomatoes, and harissa.
6. Return the eggplant to the skillet. Set the temperature on the low setting and simmer for 10 to 15 minutes.
7. Portion the millet into two dishes. Top it off with the stew. Garnish with a few leaves of cilantro and serve warm.

Nutritions: Calories: 600 Protein: 20 grams Fat: 15 grams

3. CREAMY ITALIAN WHITE BEAN SOUP

PREPARATION AND COOKINGTIME
50 MINUTES

SERVING
4 PEOPLE

INGREDIENTS

- **Vegetable oil (1 tbsp.)**
- **Onion (1)**
- **Dried thyme (.125 tsp.)**
- **Celery stalk (1)**
- **Clove of garlic (1)**
- **White kidney beans (2 - 16 oz. cans)**
- **Chicken broth (14 oz. can)**
- **Freshly cracked black pepper (.25 tsp.)**
- **Water (2 cups)**
- **Fresh spinach (1 bunch)**
- **Lemon juice (1 tbsp.)**

DIRECTIONS

1. Rinse and drain the beans.
2. Warm the oil in a large saucepan. Chop/dice the celery, garlic, and onion. Toss them into the skillet and sauté for five to eight minutes, or until tender. Mix in the garlic to sauté for 30 seconds.
3. Stir in the chicken broth, beans, pepper, two cups of water, and the thyme. Wait for it to boil and lower the temperature setting and continue cooking for 15 minutes.
4. Scoop out two cups from the soup and set it to the side.
5. Use the lowest speed on a blender to pulse/blend the rest of the soup (in batches).
6. After it is all blended, pour the soup back into the stockpot and stir in reserved beans.
7. Occasionally stir the soup as it reheats.
8. Rinse and thinly slice the spinach. Fold it in and cook it for one minute or until the spinach is wilted. away from the heat,
9. Take the pan from the burner and mix in the juice. Garnish the soup using a sprinkling of the with freshly grated Parmesan cheese.

Nutritions: Protein: 12 grams Fat: 4.9 grams Calories: 245

4. GREEK LENTIL SOUP

PREPARATION AND COOKINGTIME
1 HOUR 20 MINUTES

SERVING
4-5 PEOPLE

INGREDIENTS

- **Brown lentils (8 oz.)**
- **Olive oil (.25 cup or as needed)**
- **Minced garlic (1 tbsp.)**
- **Onion (1)**
- **Large carrot (1)**
- **Water (1 quart)**
- **Dried oregano (1 pinch)**
- **Crushed dried rosemary (1 pinch)**
- **Bay leaves (2)**
- **Tomato paste (1 tbsp.)**
- **Salt and freshly cracked pepper (as desired)**
- **Optional: Red wine vinegar (1 tsp.)**

DIRECTIONS

1. Mince the garlic and chop the onion and carrot.
2. Prep the lentils in a saucepan with enough water to cover them by about one inch. Once the beans start boiling, cook them until tender or about ten minutes, and drain in a colander.
3. Warm the oil in a skillet using the medium temperature setting. Toss in the onion, carrot, and garlic to simmer for about five minutes.
4. Pour in the water, bay leaves, lentils, oregano, and rosemary. Once it's boiling, lower the temperature setting to med-low and cover. Cook for another ten minutes.
5. Sprinkle with the pepper and salt. Stir in the tomato paste. Place a lid on the pot to simmer the soup for 30-40 minutes. Stir occasionally, adding more water as needed
6. When you are ready to serve, drizzle the soup with the vinegar and one teaspoon of olive oil.

Nutritions: Protein: 15.5 grams Calories: 357 Fat: 15.5 grams

5. PASTA FAGIOLI SOUP II

PREPARATION AND COOKINGTIME
1 HOUR 15 MIN

SERVING
8 PEOPLE

INGREDIENTS

- **Diced tomatoes (29 oz. can)**
- **Undrained Great Northern beans (2 - 14 oz. cans)**
- **Spinach (14 oz. can)**
- **Chicken broth (2 - 14.5 oz. cans)**
- **Water (3 cups)**
- **Tomato sauce (8 oz. can)**
- **Garlic (1 tbsp.)**
- **Crispy-cooked bacon (8 crumbled slices)**
- **Dried parsley (1 tbsp.)**
- **Salt (1.5 tsp.)**
- **Garlic powder (1 tsp.)**
- **Dried basil (.5 tsp.)**
- **Freshly cracked black pepper (.5 tsp.)**
- **Seashell pasta (.5 lb.)**

DIRECTIONS

1. Rinse and drain chopped spinach.
2. Prepare a large stockpot on the stovetop. Mix the beans, tomatoes, spinach, tomato sauce, chicken broth, bacon, water, minced garlic, parsley, salt, garlic powder, basil, and pepper.
3. Once it's boiling, place a top on the pot to simmer for 40 minutes.
4. Toss in the pasta (leaving the top off) and cook until its tender or for around ten minutes.
5. Serve the soup with a sprinkle cheese.

Nutritions: Calories: 256 Protein: 13.5 grams Fat: 1.1 grams

6. SWEET SAUSAGE MARSALA

PREPARATION AND COOKINGTIME
25-30 MINUTES

SERVING
6 PEOPLE

INGREDIENTS

- **Italian sausage links (1 lb.)**
- **Green and red bell pepper (1 medium of each color)**
- **Tomatoes (14.5 oz. can)**
- **Large onion (half of 1)**
- **Garlic (.5 tsp.)**
- **Dried oregano (.125 tsp.)**
- **Black pepper (.125 tsp.)**
- **Marsala wine (1 tbsp.)**
- **Water (.33 cup)**
- **Uncooked bow-tie pasta (16 oz.)**

DIRECTIONS

1. Slice the onion and green peppers. Dice the garlic.
2. Prepare a large soup pot or other pot of boiling water - about half full. Toss in the pasta and simmer for about eight to ten minutes.
3. Meanwhile, add the sausage to a medium skillet and pour in the water. Set the temperature using the med-high heat temperature. Put a top on the pot and simmer for eight minutes.
4. When the pasta is done, drain it into a colander and set it to the side for now.
5. Drain the sausage and return to the skillet. Stir in the wine, garlic, onion, and peppers. Simmer it for about five minutes using the med-high temperature setting or until done.
6. Empty in the tomatoes, oregano, and black pepper.
7. Add the pasta and continue stirring. Serve and enjoy it anytime.

Nutritions: Calories: 509 Protein: 21.9 grams Fat: 16.1 grams

7. VEGETARIAN MOROCCAN HARIRA

PREPARATION AND COOKINGTIME
1 HOUR 5 MIN

SERVING
5 PEOPLE

INGREDIENTS

- **Vegetable oil (2 tbsp.)**
- **Large onion (1)**
- **Diced tomatoes (2 lb.)**
- **Chickpeas (15 oz. can)**
- **Saffron threads (1 pinch)**
- **Fresh parsley (1 bunch)**
- **Fresh mint leaves (20 chopped leaves)**
- **Ground paprika (1 tsp.)**
- **Ground turmeric (1 tsp.)**
- **Fresh cilantro (1 bunch)**
- **Ground ginger (1 tsp.)**
- **Harissa (.5 tsp.)**
- **Water (4 cups or more to your taste)**
- **All-purpose flour (1 tbsp.)**
- **Cornstarch (1 tsp.)**
- **Cherry tomatoes (.5 cup)**
- **Salt (to your liking)**
- **Freshly cracked black pepper (as desired)**

DIRECTIONS

1. Heat the oil in a large soup pot using the medium temperature heat setting.
2. Dice and toss the onion into the pot to sauté about five minutes or until its soft and translucent.
3. Drain the chickpeas in a colander. Chop/dice the veggies and spices to your liking.
4. Dump the tomatoes, chickpeas, cilantro, parsley, mint, paprika, turmeric, ginger, harissa, and saffron. Add water and cook using medium heat until the flavors have combined or about 30 minutes.
5. Make a slurry using a few tablespoons of soup with flour and cornstarch in a mixing bowl and return it to the soup, stirring it thoroughly. Slice and add the cherry tomatoes.
6. Wait for it to boil and lower the heat setting to low.
7. Simmer until the soup thickens or approximately ten minutes and season with salt and pepper.

Nutritions: Protein: 5.7 grams Fat: 6.9 grams Calories: 182

4. MEDITERRANEAN DINNER POULTRY OPTIONS

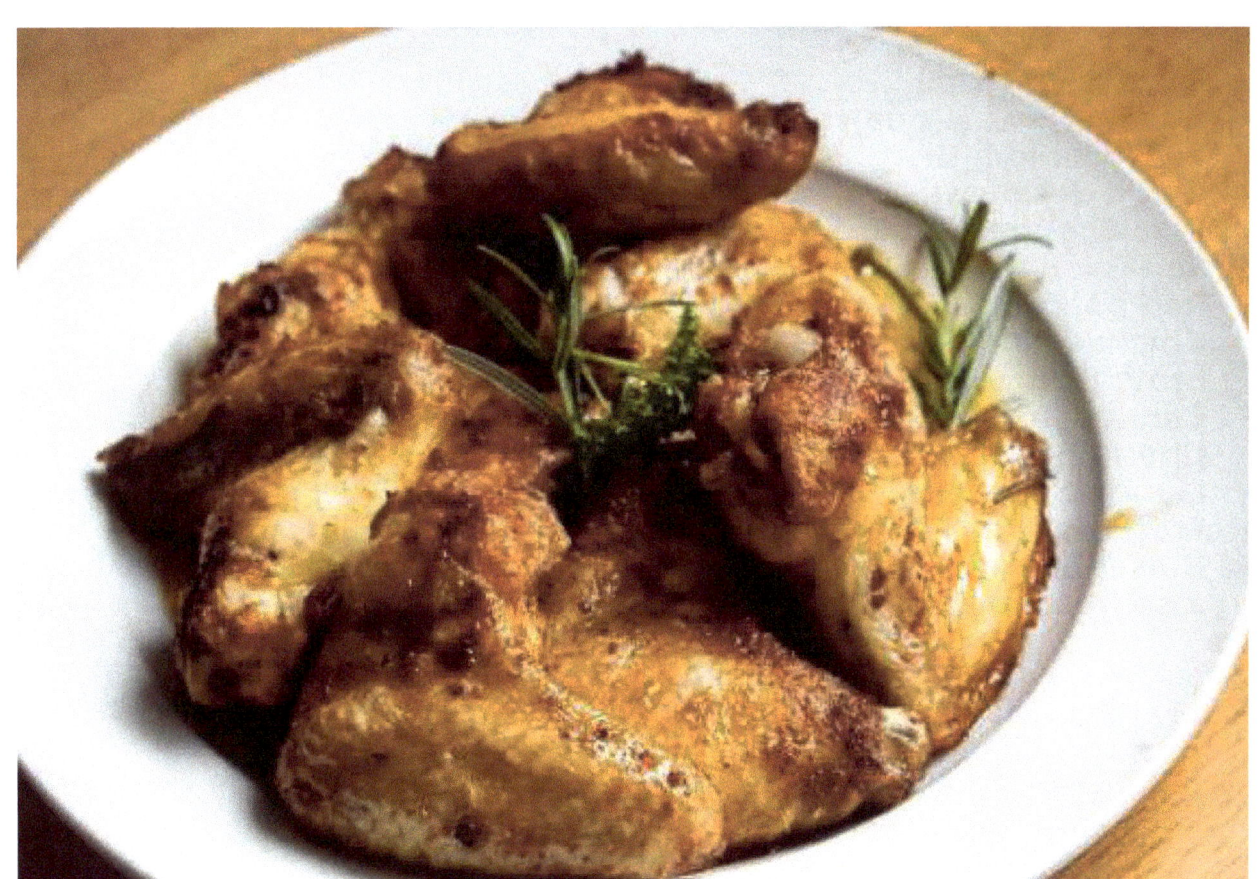

1. BRAISED CHICKEN & ARTICHOKE HEARTS

PREPARATION AND COOKINGTIME
1 HOUR 50 MIN

SERVING
4 PEOPLE

INGREDIENTS

- **Olive oil (1 tbsp.)**
- **Chicken legs (4 quarters)**
- **Yellow onion (1)**
- **Garlic (4 cloves)**
- **Black pepper (1 tbsp.)**
- **Salt (1 tsp.)**
- **Red pepper flakes (.5 tsp.)**
- **Chicken stock/low-sodium broth (1-quart)**
- **Canned artichoke hearts (10)**
- **Cherry peppers (2 cups)**
- **Lemons (2 juiced)**
- **Fresh thyme (8 sprigs)**
- **Butter beans (16 oz. can)**
- **Also Needed: Dutch oven**

DIRECTIONS

1. Dice the onion and garlic Drain thebutter beans. Drain theartichokes and cut them in half.
2. Heat the oven to reach 375° Fahrenheit.
3. Prepare the pan using the high temperature setting and add the oil.
4. Sear the chicken until browned or about five minutes per side. Set aside on a warm platter.
5. Mix in the garlic, onion, pepper flakes, salt, and black pepper Sauté it for about one minute. Stir in the broth and simmer for about a minute or so. Take the pan off of the burner.
6. Add the chicken back in the Dutch oven, adding the thyme, lemon juice, cherry peppers, and artichoke hearts.
7. Place the skillet in the oven to bake it for about one hour.
8. Take the chicken out of the cooker and place it in a warm platter again.
9. Stir the beans into the pan with the broth and artichoke mixture
10. Place each leg quarter in a serving dish. Add a ladle of the artichoke, bean, and broth mixture over each serving.

Nutritions: Calories: 707 Protein: 67.9 grams Fat: 34.9 grams

2. CHICKEN THIGHS WITH SHALLOTS IN RED WINE VINEGAR

PREPARATION AND COOKINGTIME
35 MINUTES

SERVING
4 PEOPLE

INGREDIENTS

- **Chicken thighs (32 oz. / 8 lean)**
- **Kosher salt and fresh pepper (as desired)**
- **Chicken broth (1 cup)**
- **Red wine vinegar (.5 cup)**
- **Honey (1 tbsp.)**
- **Butter (1 tsp.)**
- **Tomato paste (1 tbsp.)**
- **Shallot (1 large or .75 cup)**
- **Garlic (2 cloves)**
- **Light sour cream (2 tbsp.)**
- **Dry white wine (.5 cup)**
- **Fresh parsley (2 tbsp.)**

DIRECTIONS

1. Trim the thighs and sprinkle them using pepper and salt.
2. Prepare a medium saucepan with the honey, ¾ cup of the chicken broth, vinegar, and tomato paste. Boil until it's about ¾ cup (about 5 min.). Take the saucepan from the burner.
3. Prepare a large skillet using the med-low temperature setting. Melt the butter and add the chicken. Cook it for about six to eight minutes. Remove it and set it aside for now.
4. Thinly slice/toss the garlic and shallots into the pan. Sauté them for five minutes.
5. Pour the sauce, wine, and broth over the chicken.
6. Place a lid on the skillet, and simmer them until its tender (about 20 min.).
7. Remove the chicken and stir in the sour cream. Stir into the sauce and boil a couple of minutes.
8. Return the chicken to the skillet and garnish it with parsley.

Nutritions: Calories: 353.5 Protein: 46 grams Fat: 11.5 grams

3. FETA CHICKEN BURGERS

PREPARATION AND COOKINGTIME
30 MINUTES

SERVING
6 PEOPLE

INGREDIENTS

- **Reduced-fat mayonnaise (.25 cup)**
- **Finely chopped cucumber (.25 cup)**
- **Black pepper (.25 tsp.)**
- **Garlic powder (1 tsp.)**
- **Chopped roasted sweet red pepper (.5 cup)**
- **Greek seasoning (.5 tsp.)**
- **Lean ground chicken (1.5 lb.)**
- **Crumbled feta cheese (1 cup)**
- **Whole wheat burger buns (6 toasted)**

DIRECTIONS

1. Heat the broiler to the oven ahead of time. Combine the mayo and cucumber. Set aside.
2. Whisk each of the seasonings and the red pepper for the burgers. Work in the chicken and the cheese. Shape the mixture into six ½-inch thick patties.
3. Broil the burgers approximately four inches from the heat source. It should take about three to four minutes per side until the thermometer reaches 165° Fahrenheit.
4. Serve on the buns with the cucumber sauce. Top it off with tomato and lettuce if desired and serve.

Nutritions: Calories: 356 Protein: 31 grams Fat: 14 grams

4. GRECIAN CHICKEN & PASTA SKILLET

PREPARATION AND COOKINGTIME
40 MINUTES

SERVING
4 PEOPLE

INGREDIENTS

- **Diced tomatoes undrained - no-salt-added (14.5 oz.)**
- **Chicken broth - Reduced-sodium (14.5 oz.)**
- **Chicken breast - cut into 1-inch pieces (.75 lb.)**
- **Water or white wine (.5 cup)**
- **Garlic (1 clove)**
- **Dried oregano (.5 tsp.)**
- **Multigrain thin spaghetti (4 oz.)**
- **Marinated and quartered artichoke hearts (7.5 oz. jar)**
- **Roasted sweet bell pepper strips (.25 cup)**
- **Sliced ripe olives (.25 cup)**
- **Baby spinach (2 cups)**
- **Chopped green onion (1)**
- **Fresh parsley (2 tbsp.)**
- **Olive oil (1 tbsp.)**
- **Grated lemon zest (.5 tsp.)**
- **Lemon juice (2 tbsp.)**
- **Pepper (.5 tsp.)**
- **Optional: Crumbled reduced-fat feta cheese (as desired)**

DIRECTIONS

1. Combine the water/wine, chicken broth, chicken, garlic, oregano, and tomatoes in a large skillet. Drain and coarsely chop the artichoke hearts and add to the skillet.
2. Toss in the spaghetti and boil for five to seven minutes. Simmer it until the pink is removed from the chicken.
3. Stir in the spinach, pepper, oil, parsley, green onion, olives, red peppers, and the juice and zest of lemon.
4. Simmer for another two to three minutes or until the spinach is wilted.
5. Sprinkle it using the cheese and serve.

Nutritions: Calories: 373 Protein: 25 grams Fat: 15 grams

5. GREEK PENNE & CHICKEN

PREPARATION AND COOKINGTIME
50 MINUTES

SERVING
4 PEOPLE

INGREDIENTS

- **Skinless - boneless chicken breast halves (1 lb.)**
- **Penne pasta (16 oz. pkg.)**
- **Butter (1.5 tbsp.)**
- **Salted butter (16 oz.)**
- **Red onion (.5 cup)**
- **Cloves of garlic (2)**
- **Artichoke hearts in water (14 oz.)**
- **Tomato (1 chopped)**
- **Hunt's Diced Tomatoes (14.5 oz.)**
- **Crumbled feta cheese (.5 cup)**
- **Fresh parsley (3 tbsp.)**
- **Black pepper and salt (as desired)**
- **Lemon juice (2 tbsp.)**
- **Dried oregano (1 tsp.)**

DIRECTIONS

1. Slice the chicken into bite-sized pieces.
2. Prepare the penne until it's al dente and drain it thoroughly.
3. Melt the butter in a skillet using the med-high temperature setting.
4. Mince and toss in the garlic and onion. Sauté them for two minutes. Fold in the chicken and continue cooking for another five to six minutes.
5. Reduce the temperature setting (med-low).
6. Drain and add the artichoke hearts with the remainder of the fixings.
7. Simmer for about two to three minutes or until hot.
8. Chop the parsley and add the salt and pepper to the chicken before serving.

Nutritions: Calories: 685 Protein: 47 grams Fat: 13 grams

6. ITALIAN CHICKEN & PASTA SKILLET

PREPARATION AND COOKINGTIME
40-45 MINUTES

SERVING
4 PEOPLE

INGREDIENTS

- **Olive oil (1 tbsp.)**
- **Chicken breast halves (4)**
- **Garlic (2 cloves)**
- **Red cooking wine (.5 cup)**
- **Italian style diced tomatoes (28 oz.)**
- **Seashell pasta (8 oz.)**
- **Freshly chopped spinach (5 oz.)**
- **Shredded mozzarella cheese (1 cup)**

DIRECTIONS

1. Pour oil to a large skillet to get warm. Arrange the chicken in the pan to simmer for about five to eight minutes.
2. Pour in the diced tomatoes and wine. Wait for it to boil using the high heat temperature setting.
3. Stir in the pasta. Leave the top off and continue cooking. Stir occasionally until the shells are thoroughly cooked (approximately 10 min. after the pasta starts boiling).
4. Disperse the spinach over the top of the pasta and cover. The spinach should be ready in about five minutes.
5. Sprinkle using the cheese and simmer for another five minutes or until the cheese is bubbling.

Nutritions: Calories: 515 Protein: 43 grams Fat: 13 grams

7. LEMON CHICKEN SKEWERS

PREPARATION AND COOKINGTIME
20-25 MINUTES

SERVING
6 PEOPLE

INGREDIENTS

- **Zucchini (3 medium - 1.5-inch slices)**
- **Minced garlic (2 cloves)**
- **Medium onions (3 cut into wedges)**
- **Cherry tomatoes (12)**
- **Chicken breasts (1.5 lb.)**
- **Olive oil (.25 cup)**
- **White wine vinegar (1 tbsp.)**
- **Sugar (.5 tsp.)**
- **Lemon juice (3 tbsp.)**
- **Salt (1 tsp.)**
- **Grated lemon zest (2 tsp.)**
- **Black pepper (.25 tsp.)**
- **Dried oregano (.25 tsp.)**

DIRECTIONS

1. Slice the zucchini in half lengthwise and slice into 1.5-inch slices.
2. Peel the onions and cut them into wedges. Zest the lemon. Cut the chicken into 1.5-inch pieces.
3. Prepare the marinade. Combine the sugar, pepper, oregano, salt, lemon zest, vinegar, lemon juice, and oil - reserving .25 cup for basting. Fold in the chicken and toss to cover.
4. Add the rest of the marinade in a mixing container with the tomatoes, onions, and zucchini. Put a top or layer of plastic film/ foil over the dish and store in the refrigerator overnight (for best results) or a minimum of four hours.
5. When ready to cook, drain, and trash the marinade. Soak the wooden skewers in water.
6. Thread the chicken and veggies onto the soaked skewers.
7. Arrange the skewers on the grill for six minutes using the medium heat setting. It's done when poked with a fork - the juices will run clear.

Nutritions: Protein: 29 grams Fat: 6 grams Calories: 219

8. SLOW-COOKED MEDITERRANEAN ROASTED TURKEY BREAST

PREPARATION AND COOKINGTIME
VARIED 7,5+ HOURS

SERVING
8 PEOPLE

INGREDIENTS

- **Boneless turkey breast - trimmed (4 lb.)**
- **Chicken broth - divided (.5 cup)**
- **Fresh lemon juice (2 tbsp.)**
- **Chopped onion (2 cups)**
- **Pitted kalamata olives (.5 cup)**
- **Oil-packed sun-dried tomatoes (.5 cup)**
- **Greek seasoning - such as McCormick's (1 tsp.)**
- **Salt (.5 tsp.)**
- **Black pepper (.25 tsp.)**
- **All-purpose flour (3 tbsp.)**

DIRECTIONS

1. Thinly slice the tomatoes.
2. Arrange the turkey breast, salt, Greek seasoning, tomatoes, olives, onion, lemon juice, and ¼ cup of the chicken broth into the slow cooker. Secure the lid set the timer for 7 hours on the low setting.
3. Mix the remainder of the broth with the flour in a small mixing container. Beat/whisk until smooth and add it to the slow cooker at the end of the 7-hour cooking time.
4. Cover and c low for another 30 minutes before serving.

Nutritions: Fat: 4.7 grams Protein: 60.6 grams Calories: 333

5. MEDITERRANEAN DINNER SEAFOOD & BEEF OPTIONS

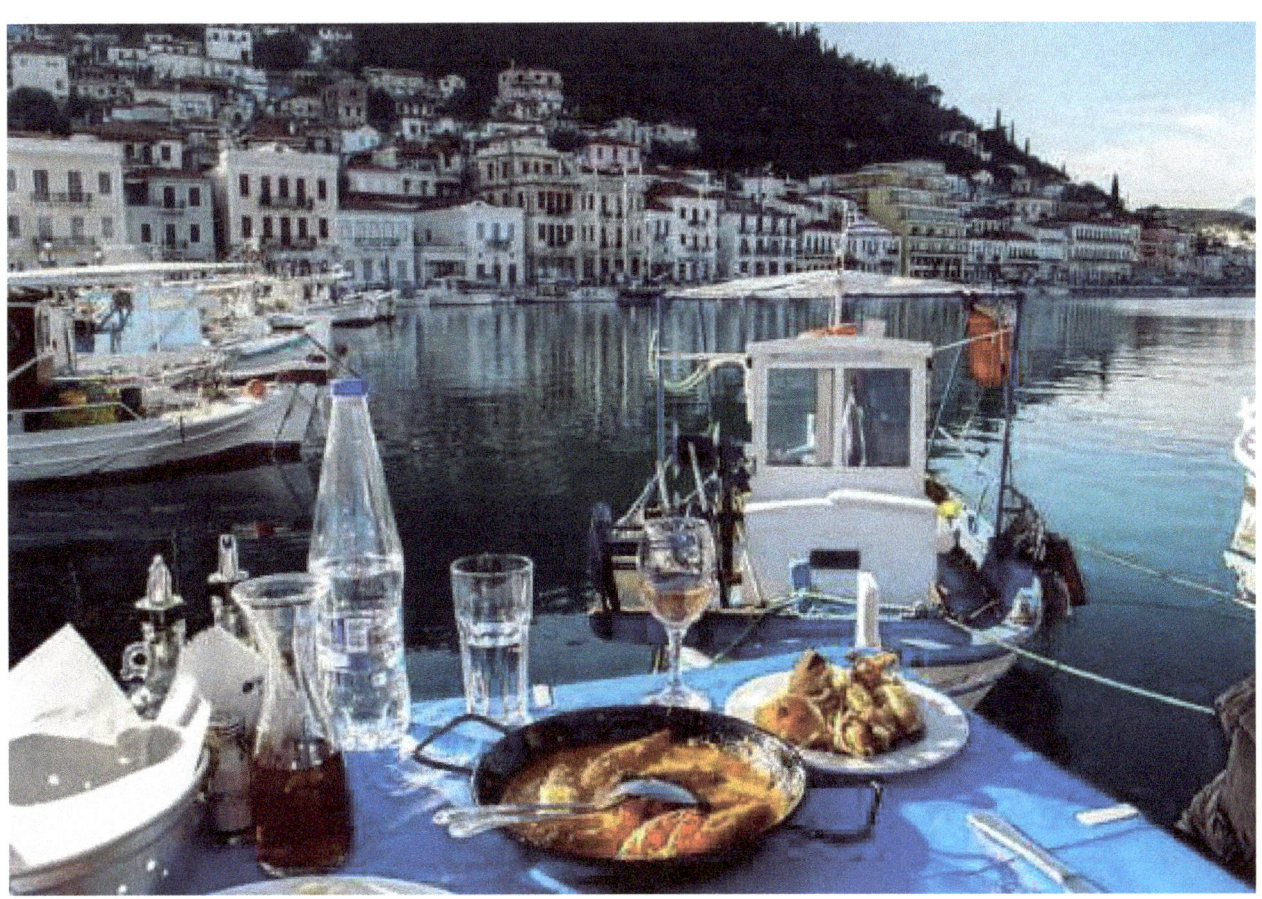

1. BAKED SALMON WITH DILL

PREPARATION AND COOKINGTIME
15 MINUTES

SERVING
4 PEOPLE

INGREDIENTS

- **Salmon fillets (4- 6 oz. portions - 1-inch thickness)**
- **Kosher salt (.5 tsp.)**
- **Finely chopped fresh dill (1.5 tbsp.)**
- **Black pepper (.125 tsp.)**
- **Lemon wedges (4)**

DIRECTIONS

1. Warm the oven in advance to reach 350° Fahrenheit.
2. Lightly grease a baking sheet with a misting of cooking oil spray and add the fish. Lightly spritz the fish with the spray along with a shake of salt, pepper, and dill.
3. Bake it until the fish is easily flaked (10 min.).
4. Serve with lemon wedges.

Nutritions: Calories: 251 Protein: 28 grams Fat: 16 grams

2. COUSCOUS WITH PEPPERONCINI & TUNA

PREPARATION AND COOKINGTIME
20 MINUTES

SERVING
4 PEOPLE

INGREDIENTS

The Couscous:
- Chicken broth or water (1 cup)
- Couscous (1.25 cups)
- Kosher salt (.75 tsp.)

The Accompaniments:
- Oil-packed tuna (2- 5-oz. cans)
- Cherry tomatoes (1 pint - halved)
- Sliced pepperoncini (.5 cup)
- Chopped fresh parsley (.33 cup)
- Capers (.25 cup)
- Olive oil (for serving)
- Black pepper & kosher salt (as desired)
- Lemon (1 quartered)

DIRECTIONS

1. Make the couscous in a small saucepan using water or broth. Prepare it using the medium heat temperature setting. Let it sit for about ten minutes.
2. Toss the tomatoes, tuna, capers, parsley, and pepperoncini into a mixing bowl.
3. Fluff the couscous when done and dust using the pepper and salt. Spritz it using the oil and serve with the tuna mix and a lemon wedge.

Nutritions: Calories: 226 Protein: 8 grams Fat: 1 gram

3. HERB-CRUSTED HALIBUT

PREPARATION AND COOKINGTIME
25 MINUTES

SERVING
4 PEOPLE

INGREDIENTS

- **Fresh parsley (.33 cup)**
- **Fresh dill (.25 cup)**
- **Fresh chives (.25 cup)**
- **Lemon zest (1 tsp.)**
- **Panko breadcrumbs (.75 cup)**
- **Olive oil (1 tbsp.)**
- **Freshly cracked black pepper (.25 tsp.)**
- **Sea salt (1 tsp.)**
- **Halibut fillets (4 - 6 oz.)**

DIRECTIONS

1. Chop the fresh dill, chives, and parsley. Prepare a baking tray using a sheet of foil. Set the oven to reach 400° Fahrenheit.
2. Combine the salt, pepper, lemon zest, olive oil, chives, dill, parsley, and the breadcrumbs in a mixing bowl.
3. Rinse the halibut thoroughly. Use paper towels to dry it before baking.
4. Arrange the fish on the baking sheet. Spoon the crumbs over the fish and press it into each of the fillets.
5. Bake it until the top is browned and easily flaked or about 10 to 15 minutes.

Nutritions: Calories: 273 Protein: 38 grams Fat: 7 grams

4. MARINATED TUNA STEAK

PREPARATION AND COOKINGTIME
15-20 MINUTES

SERVING
4 PEOPLE

INGREDIENTS

- **Olive oil (2 tbsp.)**
- **Orange juice (.25 cup)**
- **Soy sauce (.25 cup)**
- **Lemon juice (1 tbsp.)**
- **Fresh parsley (2 tbsp.)**
- **Garlic clove (1)**
- **Ground black pepper (.5 tsp.)**
- **Fresh oregano (.5 tsp.)**
- **Tuna steaks (4 - 4 oz. steaks)**

DIRECTIONS

1. Mince the garlic and chop the oregano and parsley.
2. In a glass container, mix the pepper, oregano, garlic, parsley, lemon juice, soy sauce, olive oil, and orange juice.
3. Warm the grill using the high heat setting. Grease the grate with oil.
4. Add to tuna steaks and cook for five to six minutes. Turn and baste with the marinated sauce.
5. Cook another five minutes or until it's the way you like it. Discard the remaining marinade.

Nutritions: Calories: 200 Protein: 27.4 grams Fat: 7.9 grams

5. MEDITERRANEAN FLOUNDER

PREPARATION AND COOKINGTIME
45 MINUTES

SERVING
4 PEOPLE

INGREDIENTS

- **Roma or plum tomatoes (5)**
- **Extra-virgin olive oil (2 tbsp.)**
- **Spanish onion (half of 1)**
- **Garlic (2 cloves)**
- **Italian seasoning (1 pinch)**
- **Kalamata olives (24)**
- **White wine (.25 cup)**
- **Capers (.25 cup)**
- **Lemon juice (1 tsp.)**
- **Chopped basil (6 leaves)**
- **Freshly grated parmesan cheese (3 tbsp.)**
- **Flounder fillets (1 lb.)**
- **Freshly torn basil (6 leaves)**

DIRECTIONS

1. Set the oven to reach 425° Fahrenheit. Remove the pit and chop the olives (set aside).
2. Pour water into a saucepan and bring to boiling. Plunge the tomatoes into the water and remove immediately. Add to a dish of ice water and drain. Remove the skins, chop, and set to the side for now.
3. Heat a skillet with the oil using the medium temperature heat setting. Chop and toss in the onions. Sauté them for around four minutes.
4. Dice and add the garlic, tomatoes, and seasoning. Simmer for five to seven minutes.
5. Stir in the capers, wine, olives, half of the basil, and freshly squeezed lemon juice.
6. Lower the heat setting and blend in the cheese. Simmer it until the sauce is thickened (15 min.).
7. Arrange the flounder into a shallow baking tin. Add the sauce and garnish with the remainder of the basil leaves.
8. Set the timer to bake it for 12 minutes until the fish is easily flaked.

Nutritions: Calories: 282 Protein: 24.4 grams Fat: 15.4 grams

6. MOROCCAN FISH

PREPARATION AND COOKINGTIME
1 HOUR 25 MIN

SERVING
12 PEOPLE

INGREDIENTS

- **Garbanzo beans (15 oz. can)**
- **Red bell peppers (2)**
- **Large carrot (1)**
- **Vegetable oil (1 tbsp.)**
- **Onion (1)**
- **Garlic (1 clove)**
- **Tomatoes (3 chopped/14.5 oz can)**
- **Olives (4 chopped)**
- **Chopped fresh parsley (.25 cup)**
- **Ground cumin (.25 cup)**
- **Paprika (3 tbsp.)**
- **Chicken bouillon granules (2 tbsp.)**
- **Cayenne pepper (1 tsp.)**
- **Salt (to your liking)**
- **Tilapia fillets (5 lb.)**

DIRECTIONS

1. Drain and rinse the beans. Thinly slice the carrot and onion. Mince the garlic and chop the olives. Discard the seeds from the peppers and slice them into strips.
2. Warm the oil in a frying pan using the medium temperature setting. Toss in the onion and garlic. Simmer them for approximately five minutes.
3. Fold in the bell peppers, beans, tomatoes, carrots, and olives.
4. Continue sautéing them for about five additional minutes.
5. Sprinkle the veggies with the cumin, parsley, salt, chicken bouillon, paprika, and cayenne.
6. Stir thoroughly and place the fish on top of the veggies.
7. Pour in water to cover the veggies.
8. Lower the heat setting and cover the pan to slowly cook until the fish is flaky (about 40 min.).

Nutritions: Calories: 268 Protein: 42 grams Fat: 5 grams

7. NIÇOISE-STYLE TUNA SALAD WITH OLIVES & WHITE BEANS

PREPARATION AND COOKINGTIME
20-30 MINUTES

SERVING
4 PEOPLE

INGREDIENTS

- **Green beans (.75 lb.)**
- **Solid white albacore tuna (12 oz. can)**
- **Great Northern beans (16 oz. can)**
- **Sliced black olives (2.25 oz.)**
- **Thinly sliced medium red onion (¼ of 1)**
- **Hard-cooked eggs (4 large)**
- **Dried oregano (1 tsp.)**
- **Olive oil (6 tbsp.)**
- **Black pepper and salt (as desired)**
- **Finely grated lemon zest (.5 tsp.)**
- **Water (.33 cup)**
- **Lemon juice (3 tbsp.)**

DIRECTIONS

1. Drain the can of tuna, Great Northern beans, and black olives. Trim and snap the green beans into halves. Thinly slice the red onion. Cook and peel the eggs until hard-boiled.
2. Pour the water and salt into a skillet and add the beans. Place a top on the pot and switch the temperature setting to high. Wait for it to boil.
3. Once the beans are cooking, set a timer for five minutes. Immediately, drain and add the beans to a cookie sheet with a raised edge on paper towels to cool.
4. Combine the onion, olives, white beans, and drained tuna. Mix them with the zest, lemon juice, oil, and oregano.
5. Dump the mixture over the salad and gently toss.
6. Adjust the seasonings to your liking. Portion the tuna-bean salad with the green beans and eggs to serve.

Nutritions: Calories: 548 Protein: 36.3 grams Fat: 30.3 grams

8. PAN-SEARED SALMON

PREPARATION AND COOKINGTIME
20 MINUTES

SERVING
4 PEOPLE

INGREDIENTS

- **Salmon fillets (4 @ 6 oz. each)**
- **Olive oil (2 tbsp.)**
- **Capers (2 tbsp.)**
- **Pepper & salt (.125 tsp. each)**
- **Lemon (4 slices)**

DIRECTIONS

1. Warm a heavy skillet for about three minutes using the medium heat temperature setting.
2. Lightly spritz the salmon with oil. Arrange them in the pan and increase the temperature setting to high.
3. Sear for approximately three minutes. Sprinkle with the salt, pepper, and capers.
4. Flip the salmon over and continue cooking for five minutes or until browned the way you like it.
5. Garnish with lemon slices and serve.

Nutritions: Calories: 371 Protein: 33.7 grams Fat: 25.1 grams

9. PAN-SEARED SCALLOPS WITH PEPPER & ONIONS IN ANCHOVY OIL

PREPARATION AND COOKINGTIME
45 MINUTES

SERVING
4 PEOPLE

INGREDIENTS

- **Olive oil (.33 cup)**
- **Anchovy fillets (2 oz. can)**
- **Jumbo sea scallops (1 lb.)**
- **Orange & red bell pepper (1 large of each)**
- **Red onion (1)**
- **Garlic (2 cloves)**
- **Lime zest (1 tsp.)**
- **Lemon zest (1.5 tsp.)**
- **Kosher salt & pepper (1 pinch of each)**
- **Garnish: Fresh parsley (8 sprigs)**

DIRECTIONS

1. Coarsely chop the peppers and onions. Mince the garlic and anchovy fillet. Zest/mince the lime and lemon.
2. Heat the oil and anchovies in a large skillet using a med-high temperature setting.
3. After the anchovies are sizzling, toss in the scallops, and simmer them for about two minutes - without stirring.
4. Toss the bell peppers, garlic, red onion, lime zest, lemon zest, salt, and pepper into a mixing container. Sprinkle the mixture over the scallops. Cook until they have browned (2 min.).
5. Flip the scallops, stir, and continue cooking until the scallops have browned thoroughly (4-5 min.).
6. Top it off using sprigs of parsley before serving.

Nutritions: Calories: 368 Protein: 24.2 grams Fat: 23.9 grams

10. SALMON WITH WARM TOMATO-OLIVE SALAD

PREPARATION AND COOKINGTIME
25 MINUTES

SERVING
4 PEOPLE

INGREDIENTS

- **Salmon fillets (4/approx. 4 oz./1.25-inches thick)**
- **Celery (1 cup)**
- **Medium tomatoes (2)**
- **Fresh mint (.25 cup)**
- **Kalamata olives (.5 cup)**
- **Garlic (.5 tsp.)**
- **Salt (1 tsp. + more to taste)**
- **Honey (1 tbsp.)**
- **Red pepper flakes (.25 tsp.)**
- **Olive oil (2 tbsp. + more for the pan)**
- **Vinegar (1 tsp.)**

DIRECTIONS

1. Slice the tomatoes and celery into 1-inch pieces and mince the garlic. Chop the mint and the olives.
2. Heat the oven using the broiler setting.
3. Whisk the oil, vinegar, honey, red pepper flakes, and salt (1 tsp.). Brush the mixture onto the salmon.
4. Line the broiler pan with a sheet of foil. Spritz the pan lightly with olive oil, and add the fillets (skin side downward).
5. Broil them for four to six minutes until well done.
6. Meanwhile, make the tomato salad. Mix ½ teaspoon of the salt with the garlic.
7. Prepare a small saucepan on the stovetop using the med-high temperature setting. Pour in the rest of the oil and add the garlic mixture with the olives and one tablespoon of vinegar. Simmer for about three minutes.
8. Prepare the serving dishes. Pour the bubbly mixture into the bowl and add the mint, tomato, and celery. Dust it with the salt as desired and toss.
9. When the salmon is done, serve with a tomato salad.

Nutritions: Calories: 433 Protein: 38 grams Fat: 26 grams

11. SHRIMP & PENNE

PREPARATION AND COOKINGTIME
35 MINUTES

SERVING
8 PEOPLE

INGREDIENTS

- **Penne pasta (16 oz. pkg.)**
- **Salt (.25 tsp.)**
- **Olive oil (2 tbsp.)**
- **Diced tomatoes (2 - 14.5 oz. cans)**
- **Garlic (1 tbsp.)**
- **Red onion (.25 cup)**
- **White wine (.25 cup)**
- **Shrimp (1 lb.)**
- **Grated parmesan cheese (1 cup)**

DIRECTIONS

1. Dice the red onion and garlic. Peel and devein the shrimp.
2. Add salt to a large soup pot of water and set it on the stovetop to boil. Add the pasta and cook for nine to ten minutes. Drain it thoroughly in a colander.
3. Empty oil into a skillet. Warm it using the medium temperature setting.
4. Toss in the garlic and onion to sauté until they're tender.
5. Pour in the tomatoes and wine. Continue cooking for about ten minutes, stirring occasionally.
6. Fold in the shrimp and continue cooking for about five minutes or until it's opaque.
7. Combine the pasta and shrimp and top it off with the cheese to serve.

Nutritions: Fat: 8.5 grams Protein: 24.5 grams Calories: 385

12. TILAPIA WITH AVOCADO & RED ONION

PREPARATION AND COOKINGTIME
15 MINUTES

SERVING
4 PEOPLE

INGREDIENTS

- **Olive oil (1 tbsp.)**
- **Sea salt (.25 tsp.)**
- **Fresh orange juice (1 tbsp.)**
- **Tilapia fillets (four 4 oz. - more rectangular than square)**
- **Red onion (.25 cup)**
- **Sliced avocado (1)**
- **Also Needed: 9-inch pie plate**

DIRECTIONS

1. Combine the salt, juice, and oil to add into the pie dish. Work with one fillet at a time. Place it in the dish and turn to coat all sides.
2. Arrange the fillets in a wagon wheel-shaped formation. (Each of the fillets should be in the center of the dish with the other end draped over the edge.)
3. Place a tablespoon of the onion on top of each of the fillets and fold the end into the center. Cover the dish with plastic wrap, leaving one corner open to vent the steam.
4. Place in the microwave using the high heat setting for three minutes. It's done when the center can be easily flaked.
5. Top the fillets off with avocado and serve.

Nutritions: Calories: 200 Protein: 22 grams Fat: 11 grams

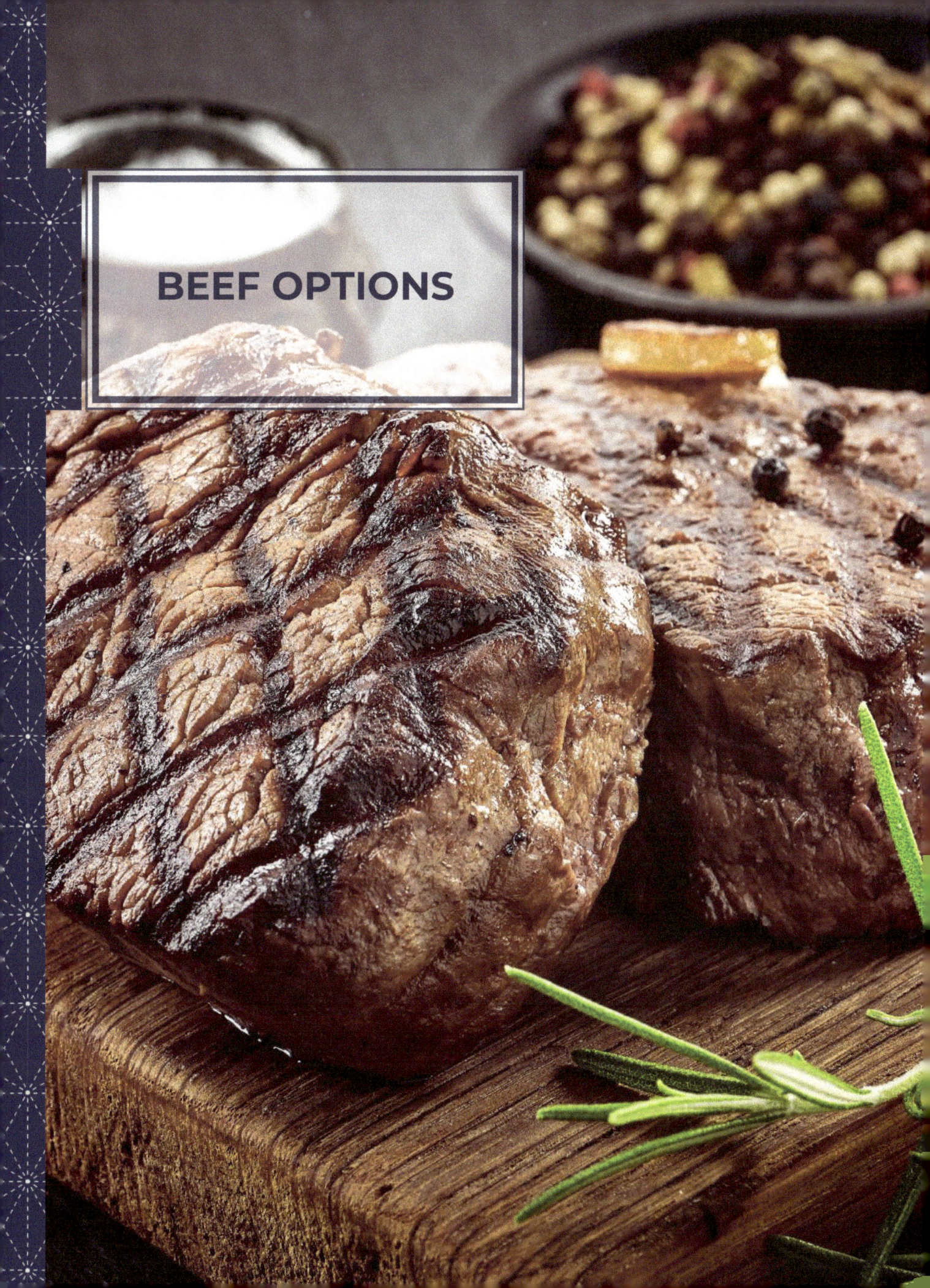

BEEF OPTIONS

1. MIXED SPICE BURGERS

PREPARATION AND COOKINGTIME
25-30 MINUTES

SERVING
6/2 CHOPS EACH

INGREDIENTS

- **Medium onion (1)**
- **Fresh parsley (3 tbsp.)**
- **Clove of garlic (1)**
- **Ground allspice (.75 tsp.)**
- **Pepper (.75 tsp.)**
- **Ground nutmeg (.25 tsp.)**
- **Cinnamon (.5 tsp.)**
- **Salt (.5 tsp.)**
- **Fresh mint (2 tbsp.)**
- **90% lean ground beef (1.5 lb.)**
- **Optional: Cold Tzatziki sauce**

DIRECTIONS

1. Finely chop/mince the parsley, mint, garlic, and onions.
2. Whisk the nutmeg, salt, cinnamon, pepper, allspice, garlic, mint, parsley, and onion.
3. Add the beef and prepare six (6) 2x4-inch oblong patties.
4. Use the medium temperature setting to grill the patties or broil them four inches from the heat source for four to six minutes per side.
5. When they're done, the meat thermometer will register 160° Fahrenheit. Serve with the sauce if desired.

Nutritions: Calories: 231 Protein: 32 grams Fat: 9 grams

6. MEDITERRANEAN DINNER PORK & LAMB OPTIONS

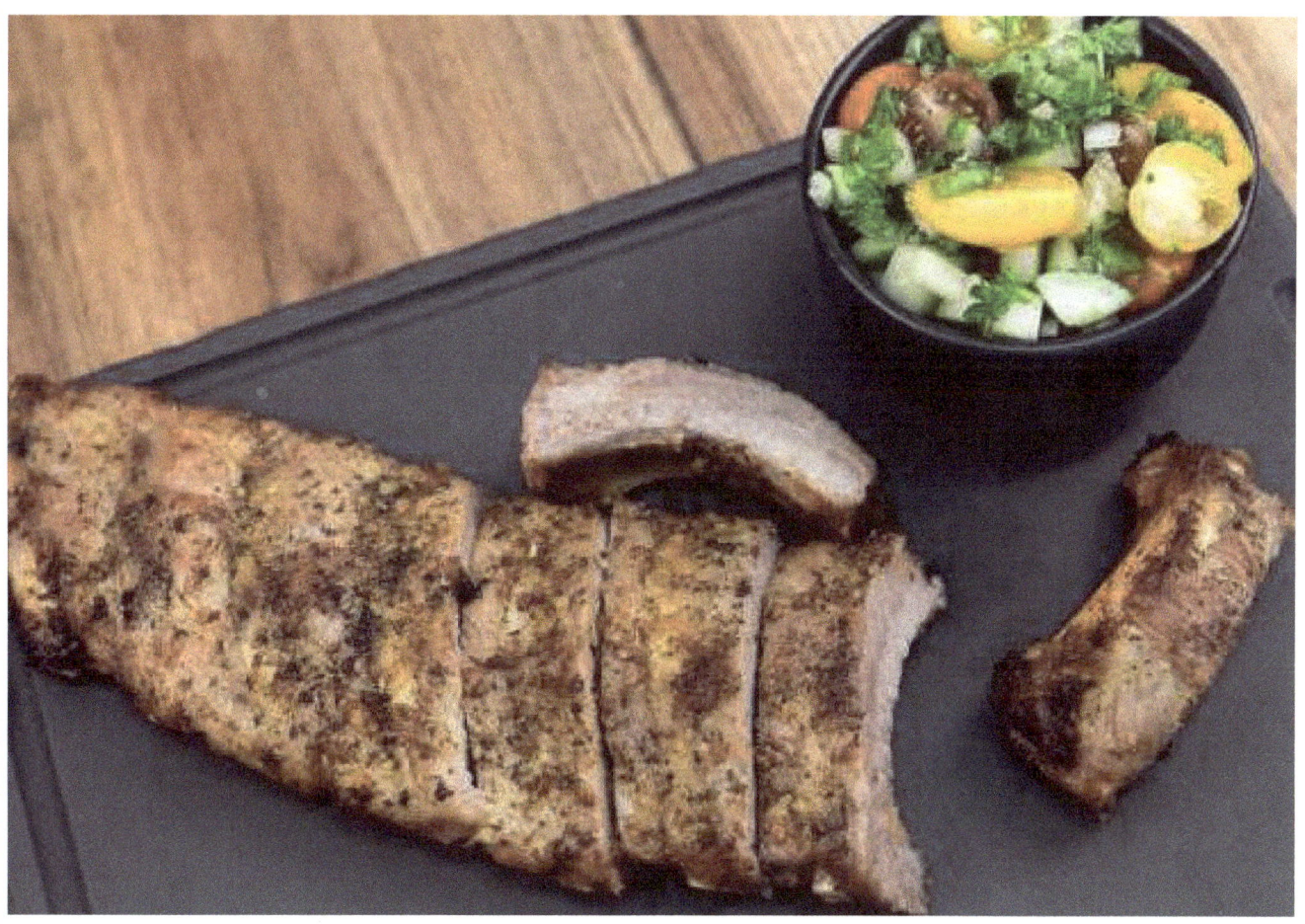

PORK FAVORITES

1. CRISPY PORK CARNITAS

PREPARATION AND COOKINGTIME
3 HOURS 55 MIN

SERVING
6 PEOPLE

INGREDIENTS

- **Olive oil (.25 cup)**
- **Boneless pork butt shoulder (3 lb.)**
- **Garlic (8 cloves)**
- **Orange (1)**
- **Kosher salt (1 tbsp.)**
- **Bay leaves (2)**
- **Black pepper (1 tsp.)**

- **Chinese 5-spice powder (.5 tsp.)**
- **Cinnamon (.75 tsp.)**
- **Ground cumin (1 tsp.)**
- **Also Needed: 9x13-inch baking dish**

DIRECTIONS

1. Set the oven to reach 275 degrees° Fahrenheit.
2. Remove all fat from the pork, slice it into two-inch cubes, and roughly chop the fat. Tear the bay leaves into halves. Mince the garlic. Juice and slice the orange peel into thin strips.
3. Mix the olive oil, pork, cinnamon, orange peel, garlic, orange juice, bay leaves, black pepper, salt, cumin, and 5-spice powder in a bowl until the pork is thoroughly covered. Dump the mixture into the baking dish.
4. Arrange the baking dish on a baking tray and cover it tightly using a layer of foil.
5. Bake until the pork is fork-tender (3.5 hrs.).
6. Arrange the oven rack about six inches. Heat the oven using the broiler.
7. Place the meat in a colander placed over a bowl. Remove bay leaves, garlic, and orange peels from the baking dish.
8. Empty the accumulated juices from the baking dish over the meat in the colander. Return the pork to the baking dish and drizzle the accumulated juices over each piece of meat.
9. Broil the pork for three minutes. Drizzle more juices over the meat and continue broiling until it's crispy (3-5 min.).
10. Transfer the pork to a serving plate with juices over the top and serve.

Nutritions: Calories: 317 Protein: 25.5 grams Fat: 22.6 grams

2. CJ'S PORCHETTA

PREPARATION AND COOKINGTIME
9 HOURS 45 MIN

SERVING
6 PEOPLE

INGREDIENTS

- **Boneless pork shoulder blade roast (2.5 lb.)**
- **Olive oil**
- **Black pepper and Kosher salt - divided (1 tbsp. each)**
- **Sage leaves (2 tbsp.)**
- **Fresh rosemary (2 tbsp.)**
- **Garlic cloves (6)**

- **Fennel seeds (2 tsp.)**
- **Orange (1 zested)**
- **Olive oil (2 tsp.)**
- **Vinegar sauce:**
- **Anchovy fillet (half of 1)**
- **White wine vinegar (.25 cup)**
- **Red pepper flakes (1 tsp.)**
- **Italian parsley (.25 cup)**

DIRECTIONS

1. Lightly crush the fennel, mince the garlic, and chop the rosemary and sage.
2. Place the roast on a cutting block to make a lengthwise (about 1 inch from th edge of the meat - but not cutting it all the way through).
3. Open the meat (using a sharp knife) flat along with the cut of the roast, so that you can unroll it into a large - flat piece.
4. Drizzle and rub the cut surface with two teaspoons of oil. Dust it using two teaspoons of black pepper, salt, sage, rosemary, orange zest, crushed fennel seeds, and garlic.
5. Push the seasonings in firmly, roll up the roast, and tie it in several places using kitchen twine.
6. Place the pork roast on a baking tray and sprinkle it using the rest of the salt (1 tsp.). Place the roast in the fridge without a covering/top overnight to dry-age.
7. Time to Bake: Set the oven temperature at 450° Fahrenheit.
8. Lightly spritz a baking dish and add the roast. Rub the meat using two teaspoons of oil.
9. Bake it in the hot oven until the outside is seared (15 min.).
10. Lower the oven temperature setting to 250° Fahrenheit. Roast until an instant read meat thermometer inserted into the center of the roast reads 145° Fahrenheit (approx. 1 hr.).
11. Loosely cover the roast with foil and wait for it to rest about ten minutes. Thinly slice it before serving.
12. Mash the anchovy fillet and mix with the white wine vinegar, red pepper flakes, and parsley.
13. Stir and scoop the mixture to drizzle it over the pork.

Nutritions: Calories: 266 Protein: 19.8 grams Fat: 19.1 grams

3. DELICIOUS PORK & ORZO

PREPARATION AND COOKINGTIME
30 MINUTES

SERVING
6 PEOPLE

INGREDIENTS

- **Pork tenderloin (1.5 lb.)**
- **Olive oil (2 tbsp.)**
- **Water (3 quarts)**
- **Uncooked orzo pasta (1.25 cups)**
- **Salt (.25 tsp.)**
- **Coarsely ground pepper (1 tsp.)**
- **Fresh baby spinach (6 oz. pkg.)**
- **Grape tomatoes (1 cup)**
- **Feta cheese (.75 cup)**

DIRECTIONS

1. Rub the pork in pepper and slice the pepper into one-inch cubes.
2. Prepare a large skillet with oil and warm using the medium temperature setting.
3. Toss in the pork and cook for eight to ten minutes.
4. Pour water and salt in a Dutch oven and wait for it to boil. Add the orzo to simmer (lid off) for eight minutes. Stir in the spinach and cook until it's wilted and tender (45-60 sec.). Drain it in a colander.
5. Cut the tomatoes into halves and add in with the pork and heat, adding in the orzo mixture and crumbled feta cheese.

Nutritions: Calories: 372 Protein: 31 grams Fat: 11 grams

4. GREEK HONEY & LEMON PORK CHOPS

PREPARATION AND COOKINGTIME
4 HOUR 20 MIN

SERVING
4 PEOPLE

INGREDIENTS

- **Pork rib chops (4)**
- **Salt (.5 tsp.)**
- **Lemon juice (2 tbsp.)**
- **Freshly trimmed mint (1 tbsp.)**
- **Honey (2 tbsp.)**
- **Cayenne pepper (.25 tsp.)**
- **Olive oil (1 tbsp.)**
- **Shredded lemon peel (2 tbsp.)**

DIRECTIONS

1. Remove all fat from the pork chops. Snip the fresh mint and shred the lemon peel.
2. Slice the chops into one-inch-thick chunks, and toss them into a large plastic zipper-type resealable bag.
3. Whisk the rest of the fixings and pour over the pork. Seal the bag.
4. Rotate the bag a few times and let it marinate for about four hours.
5. When ready to cook, prepare the grill. Grease the grilling rack with oil, and preheat the grill using the medium heat setting.
6. Arrange the chops on the grilling rack to grill for five to six minutes per side. The meat thermometer should reach 160° Fahrenheit.
7. Serve immediately.

Nutritions: Calories: 257 Protein: 29 grams Fat: 3 grams

5. MARINATED BALSAMIC PORK LOIN - SKILLET

PREPARATION AND COOKINGTIME
35 MINUTES

SERVING
4 PEOPLE

INGREDIENTS

For the Marinade:
- Pork tenderloin (1 lb. - sliced - 0.33 to 0.5-inch thickness)
- Balsamic vinegar (.25 cup)
- Olive/avocado oil (0.25 to 0.33 cup)
- Smoked/regular paprika (.5 tsp.)
- Optional: Honey (1 tbsp.)
- Minced garlic (.5 tsp.)
- Salt/pepper (.25 tsp.)
- Oregano (.25 tsp.)
- Optional 1/4 tsp dried marjoram or rosemary

For the skillet (after the pork has marinated):
- Sliced red onion (1 cup)
- Sliced olives (2 oz.)
- Zucchini (1- thinly sliced)
- Fresh basil(as preferred)
- Salt/pepper (if desired)
- To Garnish: Extra paprika or red pepper flakes
- Serve with mixed leafy greens

DIRECTIONS

1. Slice the pork and place it in a zipper-type plastic bag or inside of a large container.
2. Whisk the balsamic marinade fixings and add to pork slices.
3. Marinate them for 20 to 30 minutes in the refrigerator (longer if desired)
4. While the pork is marinating, slice the veggies.
5. Once marinated, remove and prepare a skillet using medium heat. Sauté the onion first until fragrant. No oil needed.
6. Next, add the pork loin strips and the remaining marinade sauce.
7. Cook on medium for five minutes, then flip over pork slices. Add in the olive and zucchini slices.
8. Cook it until the pork is no longer pink (five to seven minutes).
9. Plate the pork and veggies. Serve with the sauce and marinade. Top it off using fresh basil.
10. Add more paprika, salt, and pepper to your liking before serving.

Nutritions: Calories: 309 Protein: 26.2 grams Fat: 18.8 grams

6. MEDITERRANEAN PORK CHOPS

PREPARATION AND COOKINGTIME
30 MINUTES

SERVING
4 PEOPLE

INGREDIENTS

- **Boneless/bone-in pork loin chops (4 - 0.5-inch cut)**
- **Salt (.25 tsp.)**
- **Dried rosemary (1 tsp.) or fresh (1 tbsp.)**
- **Freshly cracked black pepper (.25 tsp.)**
- **Minced garlic (1.5 tsp.)**

DIRECTIONS

1. Heat the oven at 425° Fahrenheit.
2. Dust the chops using salt and pepper. Set to the side.
3. Whisk the rosemary and garlic and rub it into the chops.
4. Prepare a roasting pan with aluminum foil. Arrange the chops in it.
5. Lower the oven temperature to 350° Fahrenheit and roast it for 25 minutes. Serve right away.

Nutritions: Calories: 161 Protein: 25 grams Fat: 5 grams

7. PORK CHOPS ITALIANO

PREPARATION AND COOKINGTIME
85 MINUTES

SERVING
6 PEOPLE

INGREDIENTS

- **Olive oil (1 tsp.)**
- **Mushrooms (2 cups)**
- **Olive oil (2 tbsp.)**
- **Pork loin chops (6 - 0.75-inch thickness)**
- **Cloves of garlic (2**
- **Chopped onion (1 cup)**
- **Diced Italian tomatoes - undrained (14.5 oz. can)**
- **Basil (1 tsp.)**
- **Oregano (.5 tsp.)**
- **Freshly cracked black pepper (.25 tsp.)**
- **Salt (.5 tsp.)**
- **Water (.5 cup/as needed)**
- **Green bell pepper (1 large)**

DIRECTIONS

1. Warm one teaspoon of oil in a skillet using the medium temperature heat setting. Slice and stir in the mushrooms and sauté until they are tender (5-min.). Transfer them to a bowl and place them to the side for now.
2. Heat a skillet using the medium temperature setting to warm the rest of the oil (2 tbsp.).
3. Place the chops in the skillet to brown on both sides (7-10 min.). Put the chops on a platter. Reserve one tablespoon of drippings from the skillet.
4. Mince and stir in the garlic and onion to sauté until the onion has softened and translucent (5 min.).
5. Pour in the tomatoes, salt, pepper, basil, and oregano.
6. Place the chops back to the frying pan. Place a lid on the pot to simmer until the pork chops are fork-tender (45 min.). Add water as needed.
7. Slice the peppers into six pieces and toss them over the top of the pork, adding the reserved mushrooms.
8. Simmer until the bell pepper is tender or about 5 to 10 minutes.

Nutritions: Protein: 25.3 grams Fat: 17.6 grams Calories: 290

8. ROAST PORK FOR TACOS

INGREDIENTS

- **Pork shoulder roast (4 lb.)**
- **Diced green chilies (2 - 4 oz. cans)**
- **Chili powder (.25 cup)**
- **Dried oregano (1 tsp.)**
- **Taco seasoning (1 tsp.)**
- **Garlic (2 tsp.)**
- **Salt (1.5 tsp. or as desired)**

DIRECTIONS

1. Set the oven to reach 300° Fahrenheit.
2. Place the roast on top of a large sheet of aluminum foil.
3. Drain the chiles. Mince the garlic.
4. Mix the green chiles, taco seasoning, chili powder, oregano, and garlic. Rub the mixture over the roast and cover using a layer of foil.
5. Place the wrapped pork on top of a roasting rack on a cookie sheet to catch any leaks.
6. Roast it for 3.5 to 4 hours in the hot oven until it's falling apart. Cook until the center reaches at least 145° Fahrenheit when tested with a meat thermometer (internal temperature).
7. Transfer the roast to a chopping block to shred into small pieces using two forks. Season it as desired.

9. SLOW-COOKED PERNIL PORK

PREPARATION AND COOKINGTIME
6 HOURS 20 MIN

SERVING
6 PEOPLE

INGREDIENTS

- **Garlic (4 cloves)**
- **Large onion (1 quartered)**
- **Freshly chopped oregano (2 tbsp.)**
- **Ground ancho chile pepper (2 tsp.)**
- **Black pepper & salt (2 tsp. of each)**
- **Cumin (1 tbsp.)**
- **White wine vinegar (1 tbsp.)**
- **Boneless pork loin roast (3 lb.)**
- **Lime (1 - wedges)**
- **Olive oil (1 tbsp. or as needed)**

DIRECTIONS

1. Pulse the oregano, black pepper, onion, garlic, cumin, chile pepper, and salt in a blender, pouring in vinegar and enough olive oil until the mixture is pasty. Scrape the sides of the blender to incorporate fully.
2. Spread this mixture over the pork and add it to a slow cooker.
3. Prepare using the low setting until the pork is fork-tender (6-8 hrs.). When it's ready, cut the pork into chunks or shred.
4. Serve with a wedge of lime.

Nutritions: Calories: 367 Protein: 37.6 grams Fat: 21 grams

10. AMERICAN GYROS

PREPARATION AND COOKINGTIME
1 HOUR 55 MIN

SERVING
8 PEOPLE

INGREDIENTS

- **Ground beef & lamb (1 lb. of each)**
- **Garlic (4 cloves)**
- **Yellow onion (.5 cup)**
- **Fresh rosemary (1 tbsp.)**
- **Black pepper (1 tsp.)**
- **Kosher salt (2 tsp.)**
- **Dried oregano (2 tsp.)**
- **Cinnamon (.125 tsp.)**
- **Cumin (1 tsp.)**
- **Cayenne pepper (.125 tsp.)**
- **Paprika (1 tsp.)**
- **Dry breadcrumbs (2 tbsp.)**
- **Olive oil (1 tbsp.)**
- **Also Needed: 9x13-inch baking dish**

DIRECTIONS

1. Warm the oven at 350° Fahrenheit. Prepare the dish with a sheet of parchment baking paper.
2. Lightly oil the baking dish and paper.
3. Mix the lamb and beef in a mixing container. Dice and add the garlic, onions, salt, pepper, oregano, rosemary, cumin, cinnamon, paprika, cayenne pepper, and breadcrumbs.
4. Empty the mixture to the baking dish and press it firmly to the dish.
5. Bake in the heated oven until browned (40-45 min.). The center should read at least 160° Fahrenheit using an instant-read thermometer.
6. Cool slightly and transfer them to a platter. Cover it using a plastic wrap and refrigerate until chilled (1-2 hrs.).
7. Transfer the meat to a cutting board and cut it into three pieces - crosswise. Slice each piece into 1/8-inch thick slices as you need them.
8. Warm oil in a skillet using med-high heat. Cook the slices until browned, or about two minutes per side.

Nutritions: Calories: 255 Protein: 19.3 grams Fat: 17.8 grams

11. KOFTA KEBABS

PREPARATION AND COOKINGTIME
1 HOUR 20 MIN

SERVING
28 PEOPLE

INGREDIENTS

- **Cloves of garlic (4)**
- **Kosher salt (1 tsp.)**
- **Ground lamb (1 lb.)**
- **Grated onion (3 tbsp.)**
- **Fresh parsley (3 tbsp.)**
- **Ground coriander (1 tbsp.)**
- **Cumin (1 tsp.)**
- **Allspice (.5 tsp.)**
- **Cayenne pepper (.25 tsp.)**
- **Cinnamon (.5 tbsp.)**
- **Ground ginger (.25 tsp.)**
- **Freshly cracked black pepper (.25 tsp.)**
- **Bamboo skewers (28)**

DIRECTIONS

1. Soak the skewers for half an hour.
2. Mince and mash the garlic into a paste with the salt using a mortar and pestle. You can also use the flat side of a knife on your cutting board. Combine the garlic into the lamb along with the onion, coriander, parsley, cinnamon, cayenne pepper, allspice, ginger, and pepper in a mixing bowl.
3. Prepare the mix into the balls and flatten them into two-inch ovals.
4. Repeat the process using the rest of the skewers. Arrange the kebabs onto a baking sheet. Place in the fridge with a layer of foil or plastic. Pop them into the fridge for at least half an hour or up to 12 hours.
5. To Cook: Warm an outdoor grill using the medium temperature heat setting. Lightly spritz oil over the grate.
6. Prepare the prepared skewers, occasionally turning until the lamb has cooked (6 min. for medium).

Nutritions: Protein: 2.9 grams Fat: 2.3 grams Calories: 35

12. LAMB BOREK

PREPARATION AND COOKINGTIME
2 HOUR 5 MIN

SERVING
8 PEOPLE

INGREDIENTS

For the Lamb Filling:
- Olive oil (2 tbsp.)
- Large onion (1)
- Salt (2 tsp.)
- Ground lamb (2 lb.)
- Garlic (4 minced cloves)
- Currants (2 tbsp.)
- Toasted pine nuts (3 tbsp.)
- Ground cumin (2 tsp.)
- Cayenne pepper (.5 tsp.)
- Ground coriander (1 tsp.)
- Cinnamon (1 tsp.)
- Allspice (.25 tsp.)
- Paprika (1 tsp.)
- Freshly cracked black pepper (1 tsp.)
- Tomato sauce (1.5 cups)
- Water (.25 cup)

For the Dough:
- Large egg (1)
- Full-fat plain Greek yogurt (3 tbsp.)
- Water (2 tbsp.)
- Melted butter (2 tbsp.)
- Frozen phyllo dough, thawed (12 sheets or as needed)
- Sesame seeds (2 tsp. - optional)

For the Yogurt Sauce:
- Lemon juice (1 tsp.)
- Plain Greek yogurt (.5 cup)
- Finely sliced mint leaves (2 tbsp.)
- Clove of garlic - crushed (1 - optional)
- Water (1 tsp.)
- Salt & cayenne pepper (1 pinch)

1. Warm the oil in a saucepan using the med-high temperature setting Mince and add the onion, salt, and lamb. Break up lamb into small crumbles.
2. Cook the mixture, stirring occasionally until most of the liquid evaporates or about eight minutes. Toss in the garlic, currants, pine nuts, cumin, coriander, cinnamon, paprika, black pepper, cayenne, and allspice. Cook and stir it for one additional minute.
3. Pour tomato sauce into the lamb mixture. Add water, stir, and lower the temperature setting to medium. Continue cooking until the lamb mixture dries up, and you can stir it without seeing liquid on the bottom of the pan (20-30 min.). Turn off the heat and let cool completely before using.
4. In the meantime, combine the egg, yogurt, water, and butter in a bowl. Whisk them thoroughly.
5. Heat the oven to reach 400° Fahrenheit. Butter a round baking pan or sheet pan.
6. Place two sheets of phyllo on the work surface. Cover the rest of the sheets using a damp towel.
7. Sprinkle some egg wash lightly on top and spread using a pastry brush. Layer on two more sheets, one at a time, brushing some more egg wash over each.
8. Line ⅓ of the lamb filling along one wide edge of the phyllo. Roll the pastry, starting from the filling side, and place it against the edge of the pan. Brush more egg wash on top.
9. Shape and fill two more rolls with remaining phyllo, most of the egg wash, and filling. Wrap rolls along and inside the first one, filling the pan, and brush with egg wash. Sprinkle sesame seeds over the tops.
10. Bake in the heated oven until browned (35-40 min.). Cool it for 15 minutes.
11. Combine the yogurt, mint, lemon juice, and garlic for the yogurt sauce Mix in enough water to achieve the desired consistency for dipping Season with salt and cayenne.
12. Slice the borek into wedges and enjoy it with the sauce.

Nutritions: Calories: 449 Protein: 25.4 grams Fat: 28 grams

13. LAMB CHOPS

PREPARATION AND COOKINGTIME
30 MINUTES

SERVING
4 PEOPLE

INGREDIENTS

- **Dijon mustard (3 tbsp.)**
- **Rosemary (1 tbsp.)**
- **Garlic cloves (3)**
- **Fresh thyme (1 tbsp.)**
- **Lamb loin chops (8 - 3 oz. each)**
- **Salt (.25 tsp.)**
- **Pepper (.5 tsp.)**

DIRECTIONS

1. Mince the thyme and garlic and combine them with the mustard, garlic, rosemary, and thyme in a mixing container. Sprinkle the lamb chops using the pepper and salt.
2. Lightly grease the grill rack. Prepare the chops on the grill using the medium heat setting for six to eight minutes.
3. Note For Doneness: Medium-well is 145° Fahrenheit, the medium is 140° Fahrenheit, and well-done is at 135° Fahrenheit.

Nutritions: Calories: 231 Protein: 32 grams Fat: 9 grams

14. LAMB MEATBALLS & SAUCE

PREPARATION AND COOKINGTIME
1 HOUR 50 MIN

SERVING
4 PEOPLE

INGREDIENTS

- **Dry breadcrumbs (.5 cup)**
- **Milk (.5 cup)**
- **Egg (1 beaten)**
- **Ground lamb (1.25 lb.)**
- **Garlic cloves (3)**
- **Olive oil (2 tbsp.)**
- **Tomato paste (1 tbsp.)**
- **Fresh rosemary (1 tbsp.)**
- **Cumin (1 tbsp.)**
- **Salt (1.5 tsp.)**
- **Dried oregano (1 tsp.)**
- **Black pepper (.5 tsp.)**
- **Cinnamon (.25 tsp.)**
- **Cayenne pepper (1 pinch)**
- **Chicken stock (1 cup)**
- **Tomato sauce (3 cups)**
- **Freshly chopped mint (2 tbsp.)**
- **Red pepper flakes (1 pinch)**

DIRECTIONS

1. Warm the oven to 450° Fahrenheit.
2. Mince the garlic and chop the rosemary. Prepare a baking tray using a sheet of foil, and mist it with oil.
3. Mix the breadcrumbs and milk in a small mixing bowl. Soak them until the milk is absorbed (30 min.).
4. Combine the breadcrumb mixture, egg, lamb, garlic, tomato paste, olive oil, rosemary, cumin, salt, oregano, cinnamon, black pepper, and cayenne pepper in a large mixing container.
5. Shape the lamb mixture into two-inch meatballs and arrange them on the baking tray.
6. Prepare the meatballs in the hot oven until they are slightly browned, or (15 min.). Transfer them to the countertop for now.
7. Combine the chicken stock, tomato sauce, meatballs, pepper flakes, and fresh mint in a large saucepan using the medium temperature heat setting (45 min.). The pink should be removed when they are thoroughly done.minutes per side.

Nutritions: Calories: 610 Protein: 31.3 grams Fat: 43.5 grams

7. MEDITERRANEAN BREAD - FLATBREAD & PIZZAS

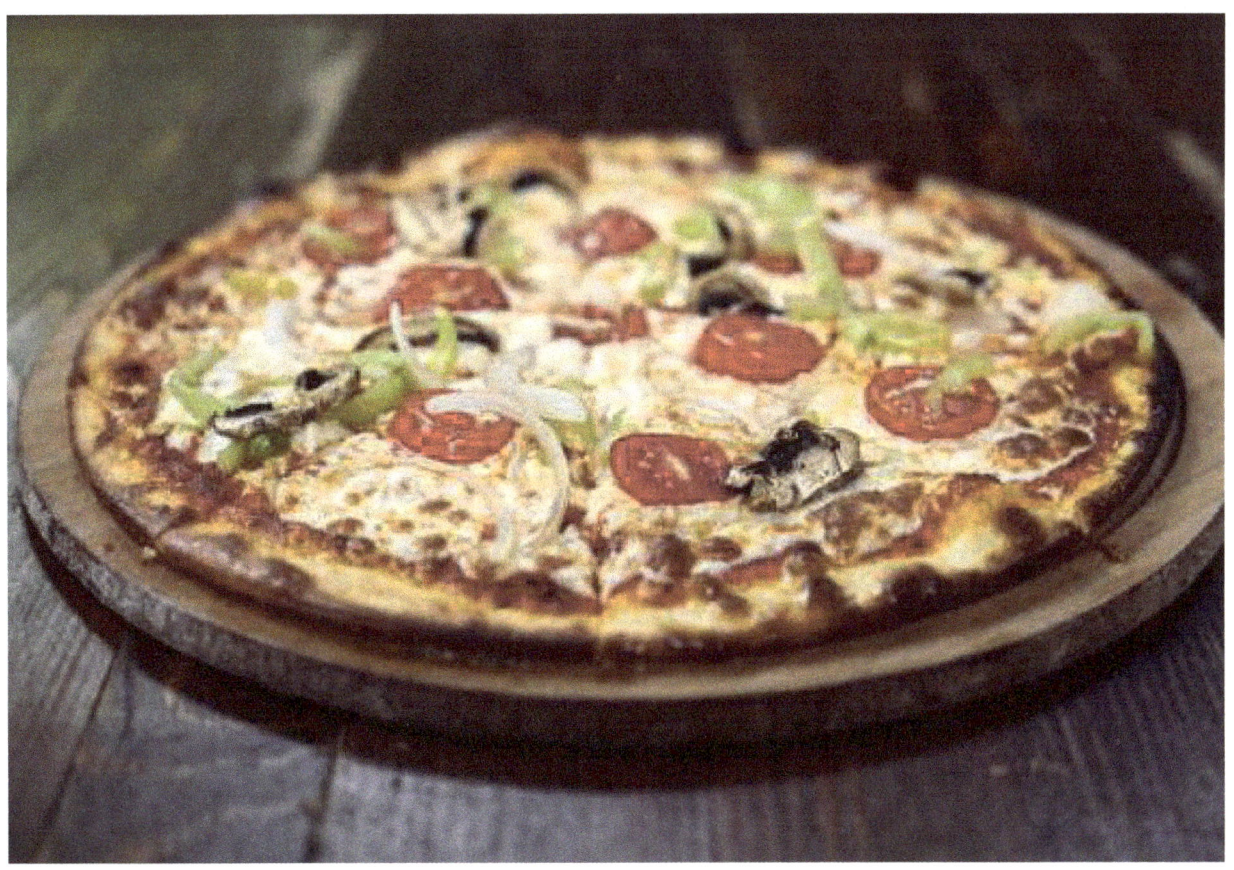

BREAD CHOICES

1. BANANA SOUR CREAM BREAD

PREPARATION AND COOKINGTIME
1 HOURS 10 MIN

SERVING
32 PEOPLE

INGREDIENTS

- **White sugar (.25 cup)**
- **Cinnamon (1 tsp.+ 2 tsp.)**
- **Butter (.75)**
- **White sugar (3 cups)**
- **Eggs (3)**
- **Very ripe bananas, mashed (6)**
- **Sour cream (16 oz. container)**
- **Vanilla extract (2 tsp.)**
- **Salt (.5 tsp.)**
- **Baking soda (3 tsp.)**
- **All-purpose flour (4.5 cups)**
- **Optional: Chopped walnuts (1 cup)**
- **Also Needed: 4 - 7 by 3-inch loaf pans**

DIRECTIONS

1. Set the oven to reach 300°Fahrenheit. Grease the loaf pans.
2. Sift the sugar and one teaspoon of the cinnamon. Dust the pan with the mixture.
3. Cream the butter with the rest of the sugar. Mash the bananas with the eggs, cinnamon, vanilla, sour cream, salt, baking soda, and the flour. Toss in the nuts last.
4. Dump the mixture into the pans. Bake it for one hour. Test for doneness with a toothpick in the center. It's done when it comes out clean.

Nutritions: Calories: 263 Protein: 3.7 grams Fat: 10.4 grams

2. HOMEMADE PITA BREAD

PREPARATION AND COOKINGTIME
5 HOURS

SERVING
7 PEOPLE

INGREDIENTS

- **Dried yeast (.25 oz.)**
- **Sugar (.5 tsp.)**
- **Bread flour /mixture of all-purpose & whole wheat (2.5**
- **cups + more for dusting)**
- **Salt (.5 tsp.)**
- **Water (.25 cup or as needed)**
- **Oil as needed**

DIRECTIONS

1. Dissolve the yeast and sugar in ¼ of a cup lukewarm water in a small mixing container. Wait for about 15 minutes (ready when it's frothy).
2. In another container, sift the flour and salt.
3. Dig a hole in the center and add the yeast mixture (+) one cup of water. Knead the mixture into a pliable dough.
4. Dump the dough onto a lightly floured surface and knead it is smooth and elastic.
5. Pour a drop of oil into the bottom of a large bowl and roll the dough in it to cover the surface.
6. Place a dampened tea towel over the container of dough. Cover the bowl with a damp cloth and place it in a warm spot for at least two hours or overnight. (The dough will double its size).
7. Punch the dough down and knead the bread and divide it into small balls. Flatten the balls into thick oval discs.
8. Dust a tea towel using the flour and place the oval discs on top, leaving enough room to expand between them. Dust with flour and lay another clean cloth on top. Let it rise for another one to two hours.
9. Set the oven at 425° Fahrenheit. Place several baking sheets in the oven to heat briefly. Lightly grease the warmed baking sheets with oil and place the oval bread discs on them.
10. Sprinkle the ovals lightly with water, and bake until they are lightly browned or for six to eight minutes. (Pitas should rise so that they are slightly hollow inside.)
11. Serve them while they are warm. Arrange the flatbread on a wire rack and wrap them in a clean, dry cloth to keep soft for later.

Nutritions: Protein: 6 grams Fat: 4 grams Calories: 210

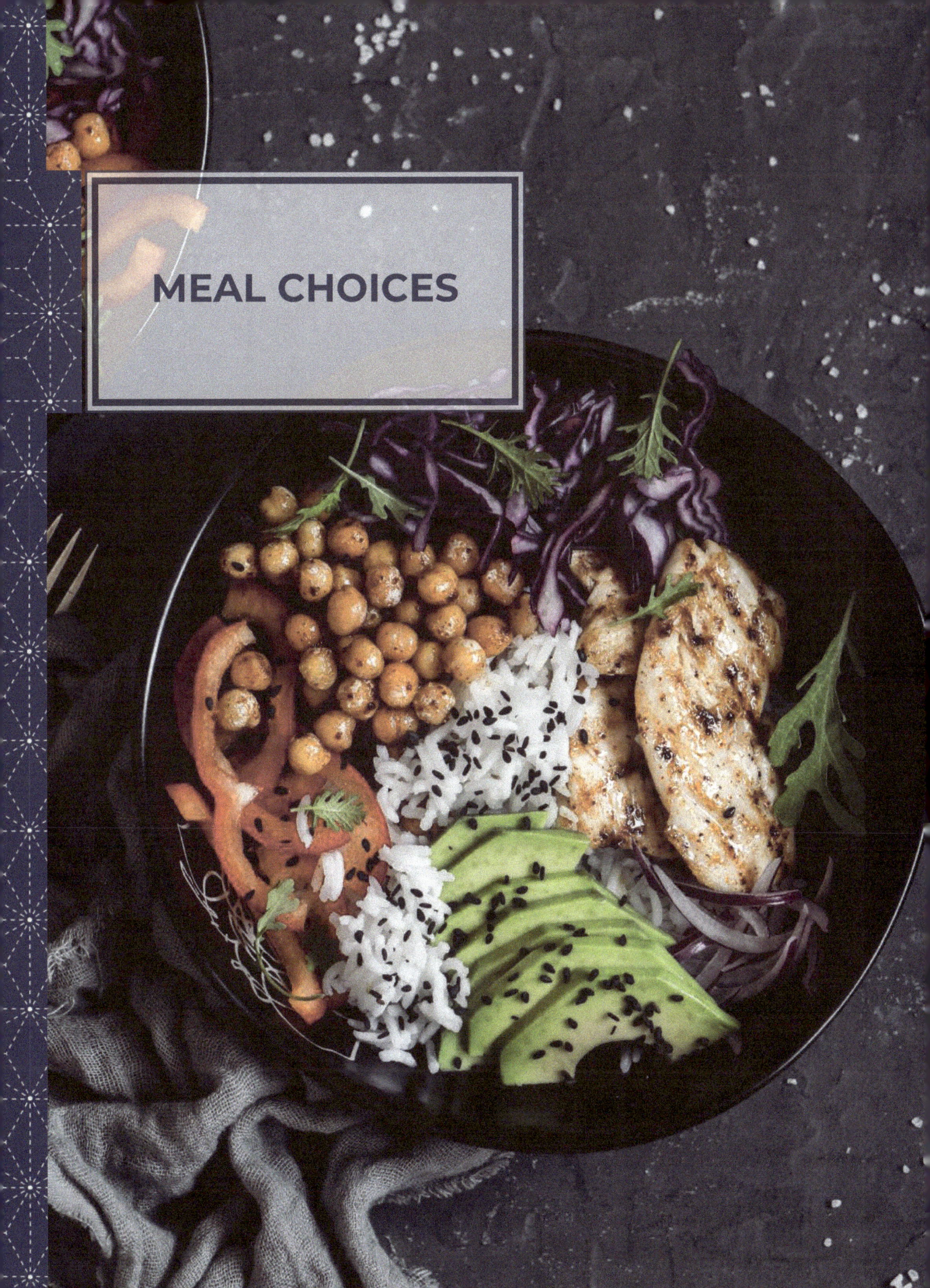

MEAL CHOICES

1. FLATBREAD SANDWICHES

PREPARATION AND COOKINGTIME
20 MIN

SERVING
6 PEOPLE

INGREDIENTS

- **Olive oil (1 tbsp.)**
- **7-Grain pilaf (8.5 oz. pkg.)**
- **English seedless cucumber (1 cup)**
- **Seeded tomato (1 cup)**
- **Crumbled feta cheese (.25 cup)**
- **Fresh lemon juice (2 tbsp.)**
- **Freshly cracked black pepper (.25 tsp.)**
- **Plain hummus (7 oz. container)**
- **Whole grain white flatbread wraps (3 @ 2.8 oz. each)**

DIRECTIONS

1. Cook the pilaf as directed on the package instructions and cool.
2. Chop and combine the tomato, cucumber, cheese, oil, pepper, and lemon juice. Fold in the pilaf.
3. Prepare the wraps with the hummus on one side. Spoon in the pilaf and fold.
4. Slice into a sandwich and serve.

Nutritions: Calories: 310 Protein: 10 grams Fat: 9 grams

2. MEZZE PLATTER WITH TOASTED ZA'ATAR PITA BREAD

PREPARATION AND COOKINGTIME
10 MINUTES

SERVING
4 PEOPLE

INGREDIENTS

- **Whole-wheat pita rounds (4)**
- **Olive oil (4 tbsp.)**
- **Za'atar (4 tsp.)**
- **Greek yogurt (1 cup)**
- **Black pepper & Kosher salt (to your liking)**
- **Hummus (1 cup)**
- **Marinated artichoke hearts (1 cup)**
- **Assorted olives (2 cups)**
- **Sliced roasted red peppers (1 cup)**
- **Cherry tomatoes (2 cups)**
- **Salami (4 oz.)**

DIRECTIONS

1. Use the medium-high heat setting to heat a large skillet.
2. Lightly brush the pita bread with the oil on each side and add the za'atar for seasoning.
3. Prepare in batches by adding the pita into a skillet and toasting until browned. It should take about two minutes on each side. Slice each of the pitas into quarters.
4. Season the yogurt with pepper and salt.
5. To assemble, divide the potatoes and add the hummus, yogurt, artichoke hearts, olives, red peppers, tomatoes, and salami. inutes per side.

Nutritions: Calories: 731 Protein: 26 grams Fat: 48 grams

3. MINI CHICKEN SHAWARMA

PREPARATION AND COOKINGTIME
1 HOUR 15 MIN

SERVING
8 PEOPLE

INGREDIENTS

- **The Chicken:**
- **Chicken tenders (1 lb.)**
- **Olive oil (.25 cup)**
- **Lemon - zest & juice (1)**
- **Cumin (1 tsp.)**
- **Garlic powder (2 tsp.)**
- **Smoked paprika (.5 tsp.)**
- **Coriander (.75 tsp.)**
- **Freshly ground black pepper (1 tsp.)**

The Sauce:
- **Greek yogurt (1.25 cups)**
- **Lemon juice (1 tbsp.)**
- **Grated garlic clove (1)**
- **Freshly chopped dill (2 tbsp.)**
- **Black pepper (.125 tsp/to taste)**
- **Kosher salt (as desired)**
- **Chopped fresh parsley (.25 cup)**
- **Red onion (half of 1)**
- **Romaine lettuce (4 leaves)**
- **English cucumber (half of 1)**
- **Tomatoes (2)**
- **Mini pita bread (16)**

DIRECTIONS

1. Toss the chicken into a zipper-type baggie. Whisk the chicken fixings and add it to the bag to marinate for up to an hour.
2. Prepare the sauce by combining the juice, garlic, and yogurt in a mixing container. Stir in the dill, parsley, pepper, and salt. Place in the fridge.
3. Heat a skillet using the medium temperature heat setting. Transfer the chicken from the marinade (let the excess drip off).
4. Cook until thoroughly cooked or about four minutes per side. Chop it into bite-sized strips.
5. Thinly slice the cucumber and onion. Shred the lettuce and chop the tomatoes. Assemble and add to the pitas - the chicken, lettuce, onion, tomato, and cucumber.

Nutritions: Calories: 216 Protein: 9 grams Fat: 16 grams

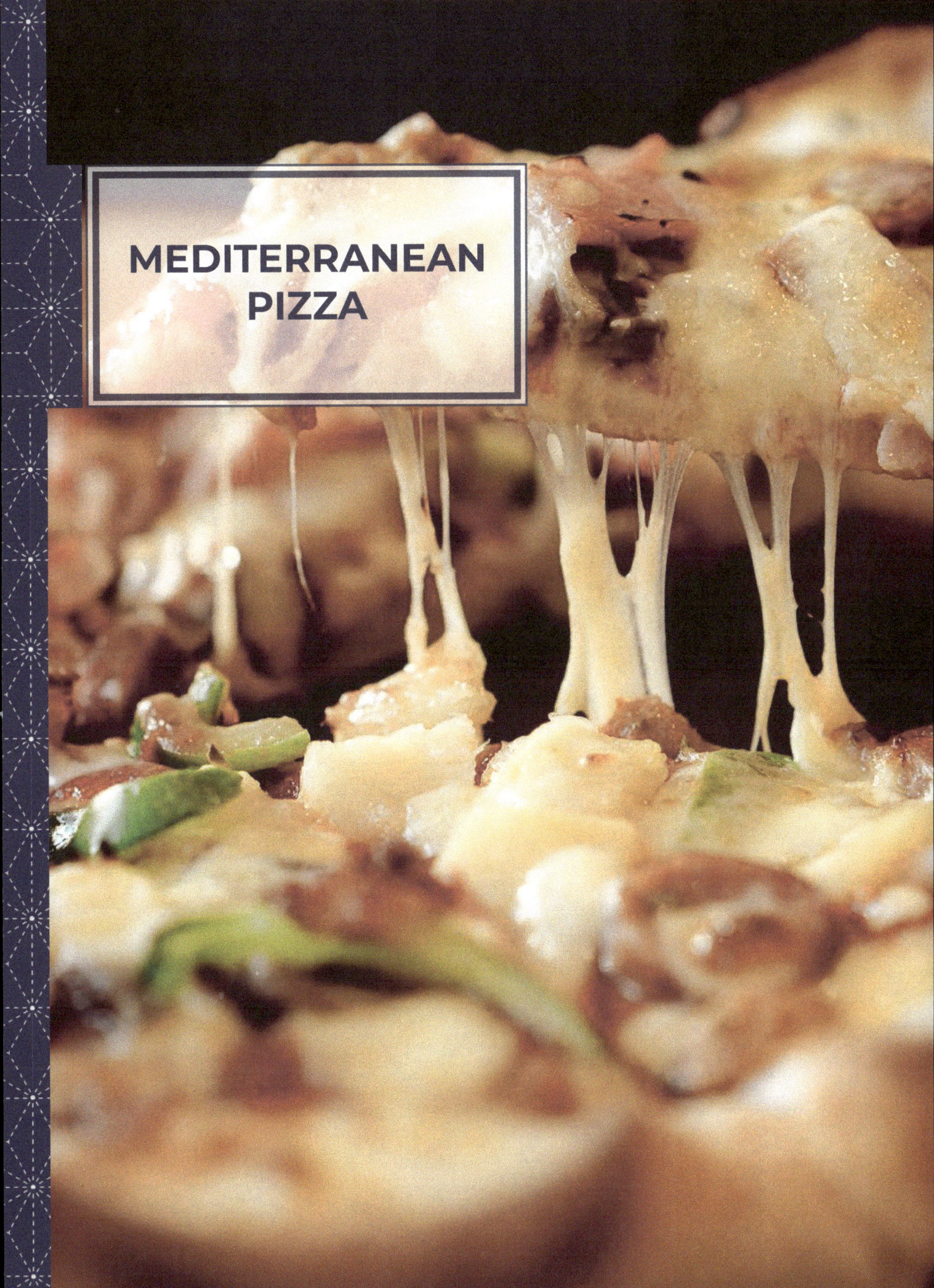

MEDITERRANEAN PIZZA

1. EGGPLANT PIZZA

PREPARATION AND COOKINGTIME
30 MINUTES

SERVING
6 PEOPLE

INGREDIENTS

- **Eggplants (1 large or 2 medium)**
- **Olive oil (.33 cup)**
- **Black pepper & salt (as desired)**
- **Marinara sauce - store-bought/homemade (1.25 cups)**
- **Shredded mozzarella cheese (1.5 cups)**
- **Cherry tomatoes (2 cups - halved)**
- **Torn basil leaves (.5 cup)**

DIRECTIONS

1. Heat the oven to reach 400° Fahrenheit. Prepare a baking sheet with a layer of parchment baking paper.
2. Slice the end/ends off of the eggplant and them it into ¾-inch slices. Arrange the slices on the prepared sheet and brush both sides with olive oil. Dust with pepper and salt to your liking.
3. Roast the eggplant until tender (10 to 12 min.).
4. Transfer the tray from the oven and add two tablespoons of sauce on top of each section. Top it off with the mozzarella and three to five tomato pieces on top.
5. Bake it until the cheese is melted. The tomatoes should begin to blister in about five to seven more minutes.
6. Take the tray from the oven. Serve hot and garnish with a dusting of basil.

Nutritions: Protein: 8 grams Fat: 20 grams Calories: 257

2. MEDITERRANEAN WHOLE WHEAT PIZZA

PREPARATION AND COOKINGTIME
25 MINUTES

SERVING
4 PEOPLE

INGREDIENTS

- **Whole-wheat pizza crust (1)**
- **Basil pesto (4 oz. jar)**
- **Artichoke hearts (.5 cup)**
- **Kalamata olives (2 tbsp.)**
- **Pepperoncini (2 tbsp. drained)**
- **Feta cheese (.25 cup)**

DIRECTIONS

1. Program the oven to 450° Fahrenheit.
2. Drain and pull the artichokes to pieces. Slice/chop the pepperoncini and olives.
3. Arrange the pizza crust onto a floured work surface and cover it using pesto. Arrange the artichoke, pepperoncini slices, and olives over the pizza. Lastly, crumble and add the feta.
4. Bake in the hot oven until the cheese has melted, and it has a crispy crust or 10-12 minutes.

Nutritions: Calories: 277 Protein: 9.7 grams Fat: 18.6 grams

3. SPINACH & FETA PITA BAKE

PREPARATION AND COOKINGTIME
22 MINUTES

SERVING
6 PEOPLE

INGREDIENTS

- **Sun-dried tomato pesto (6 oz. tub)**
- **Roma - plum tomatoes (2 chopped)**
- **Whole-wheat pita bread (Six 6-inch)**
- **Spinach (1 bunch)**
- **Mushrooms (4 sliced)**
- **Grated Parmesan cheese (2 tbsp.)**
- **Crumbled feta cheese (.5 cup)**
- **Olive oil (3 tbsp.)**
- **Black pepper (as desired)**

DIRECTIONS

1. Set the oven at 350° Fahrenheit.
2. Spread the pesto onto one side of each pita bread and arrange them onto a baking tray (pesto-side up).
3. Rinse and chop the spinach. Top the pitas with spinach, mushrooms, tomatoes, feta cheese, pepper, Parmesan cheese, pepper, and a drizzle of oil.
4. Bake in the hot oven until the pita bread is crispy (12 min.). Slice the pitas into quarters.

Nutritions: Calories: 350 Protein: 11.6 grams Fat: 17.1g rams

4. WATERMELON FETA & BALSAMIC PIZZA

PREPARATION AND COOKINGTIME
15 MINUTES

SERVING
4 PEOPLE

INGREDIENTS

- **Watermelon (1-inch thick from the center)**
- **Crumbled feta cheese (1 oz.)**
- **Sliced Kalamata olives (5-6)**
- **Mint leaves (1 tsp.)**
- **Balsamic glaze (.5 tbsp.)**

DIRECTIONS

1. Slice the widest section of the watermelon in half. Then, slice each half into four wedges.
2. Serve on a round pie dish like a pizza round and cover with the olives, cheese, mint leaves, and glaze.

Nutritions: Protein: 2 grams Fat: 3 grams Calories: 90

8. DESSERTS - FRUITY TREATS & MORE

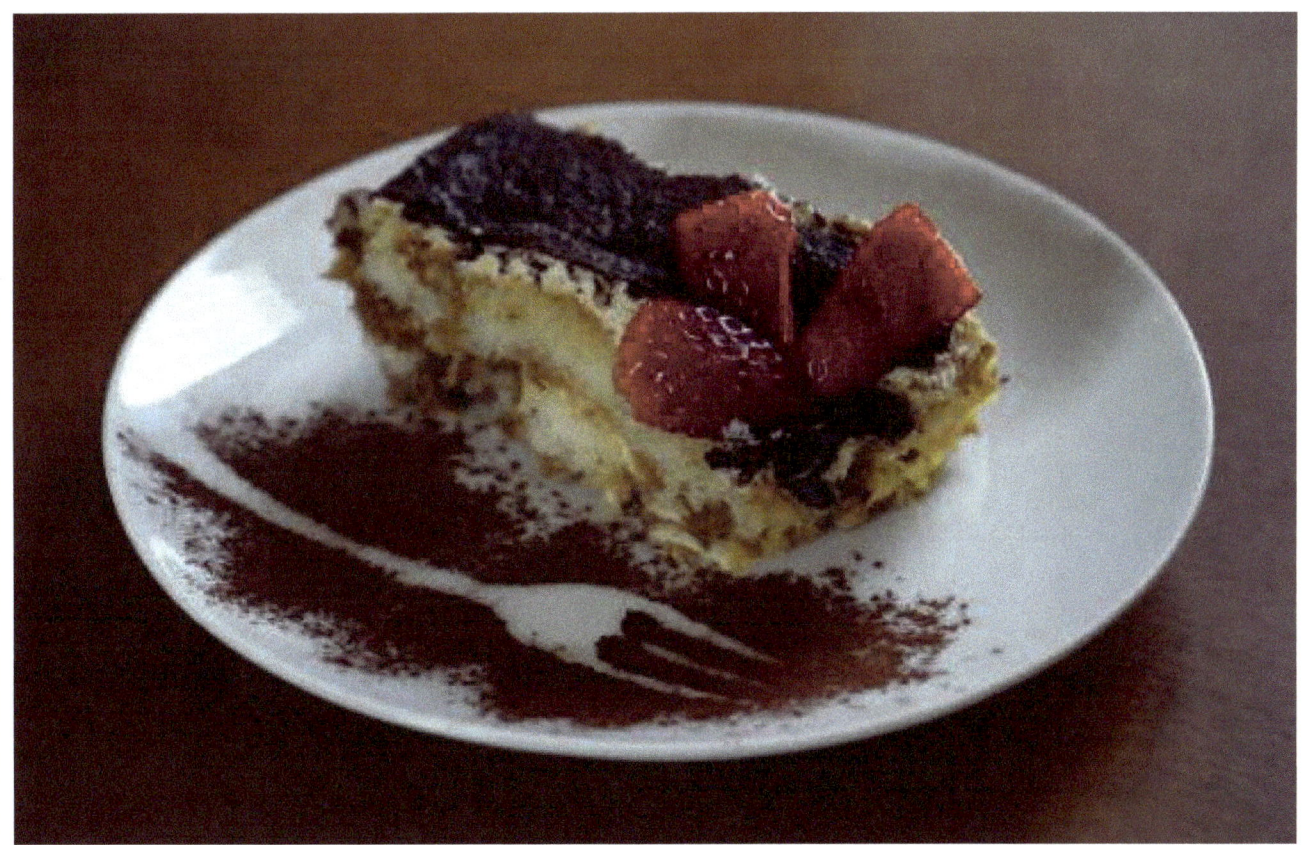

1. AVOCADO - CHOCOLATE PUDDING WITH HAZELNUTS & SEA SALT

PREPARATION AND COOKINGTIME
5 MINUTES

SERVING
4 PEOPLE

INGREDIENTS

- Chilled avocado (2 large)
- Full-fat coconut milk (.5 cup)
- Raw cacao powder (.33 cup)
- Maple syrup (.33 cup)
- Vanilla extract (2 tsp.)

The Topping:
- Roughly chopped hazelnuts
- Sea salt

DIRECTIONS

1. Use a sharp knife to slice the avocado in half and discard the pit.
2. Remove and add the flesh into a food processor and add the rest of the fixings.
3. Blend until smooth, scraping the sides as needed.
4. Serve the pudding with a sprinkle of hazelnuts and sea salt.

Nutritions: Calories: 295 Protein: 3.4 grams Fat: 20.9 grams

2. CHILLED DARK CHOCOLATE FRUIT KEBABS

PREPARATION AND COOKINGTIME
30 MINUTES

SERVING
6 PEOPLE

INGREDIENTS

- **Hulled strawberries (12)**
- **Green or red seedless grapes (24)**
- **Pitted cherries (12)**
- **Blueberries (24)**
- **Dark chocolate (8 oz.)**
- **Also Needed: 12-inch skewers (6)**

DIRECTIONS

1. Prepare a rimmed baking sheet with a sheet of parchment baking paper. Prepare the skewers with the fruit, alternating each flavor.
2. Use a microwave-safe dish to heat the chocolate on high for one minute. Stir to melt the chocolate and add it to a plastic sandwich bag and twist a corner. Snip the corner off of the bag to use as a piping device. Squeeze the bag to drizzle the chocolate over the kebabs.
3. Arrange the sheet in the freezer to chill for 20 minutes before serving.

Nutritions: Calories: 254 Protein: 3 grams Fat: 15 grams

3. CHOCOLATE ALMOND BUTTER FRUIT DIP

PREPARATION AND COOKINGTIME
15 MINUTES

SERVING
14 PEOPLE

INGREDIENTS

- **Plain Greek yogurt (1 cup)**
- **Almond butter (.5 cup)**
- **Chocolate-hazelnut spread (.33 cup)**
- **Honey (1 tbsp.)**
- **Vanilla (1 tsp.)**
- **Fresh fruit - Ex. Bananas, apples, pears, etc.**

DIRECTIONS

1. Combine all of the fixings except for the fruit of choice.
2. Whisk well or place in a blender for a creamier result.
3. Serve with the freshly sliced fruit (not included in macros).

Nutritions: Protein: 4 grams Fat: 8 grams Calories: 115

4. GREEK COCONUT CAKE WITH SYRUP

PREPARATION AND COOKINGTIME
40 MINUTES

SERVING
8-10 PEOPLE

INGREDIENTS

- Eggs (4 separated)
- Salt (1 pinch)
- Margarine/butter - softened (0.33 lb. or 0.66 cup)
- Sugar (1 cup)
- Whole milk (.5 cup)
- Self-rising flour (1.5 cups)
- Baking powder (1 tbsp.)
- Shredded coconut (1.5 cups)

For the Syrup:
- Water (2.5 cups)
- Sugar (1.5 cups)
- Lemon juice (1 tbsp.)
- Whole cloves (3)
- Lemon zest (.5 tbsp.)
- Stick of cinnamon (1)
- Butter/Margarine - for baking pan (1 tbsp.)
- Flour - needed for the baking pan (2 tbsp.)

DIRECTIONS

1. Combine each of the syrup fixings in a saucepan to boil for seven to eight minutes. Transfer the pan from the burner and set it aside to cool.
2. Warm the oven at 340° Fahrenheit.
3. Whisk the egg whites with salt to form the stiff peak stage.
4. In a separate mixing container, whisk the egg yolks, sugar, and margarine, until it's smooth and mix in milk.
5. Whisk the baking powder and flour and beat into the mixture Stir in the coconut.
6. Lastly, fold in the whisked egg whites.
7. Lightly grease a 15x10-inch baking pan with butter. Lightly coat it with flour, shaking the pan, discarding the excess flour.
8. Transfer the cake batter to the pan. Bake at 340° Fahrenheit until it's golden, and the cake starts to pull away from the sides of the pan (40-45 min.).
9. Remove the pan from the oven, cut it into pieces, and while it's hot - pour the cooled syrup evenly over the cake. Begin around the edges and move it to the center.
10. Sprinkle the top with 4 to 5 tablespoons of shredded coconut.
11. Wait for two to three hours before serving so the cake can absorb the deliciousness.

Nutritions: Calories: 479 Protein: 6 grams Fat: 23 grams

5. GREEK SEMOLINA CAKE WITH ORANGE SYRUP - REVANI

PREPARATION AND COOKINGTIME
65 MINUTES

SERVING
15 PEOPLE

INGREDIENTS

- Flour (1 cup)
- Baking powder (1 tbsp.)
- Fine semolina (1 cup)
- Unsalted butter (0.5 cup/1 stick)
- Sugar (1 cup)
- Eggs (3 separated)
- Milk (1 cup)
- Vanilla extract (1 tsp.)
- Zest of 1 lemon
- Sugar (1.5 cups)
- Salt (1 pinch)
- Water (1.5 cups)
- Two 3-inch strips of orange zest
- Fresh lemon juice (1 tsp.)

Optional:
- Ground cinnamon
- Powdered sugar
- Almonds - blanched - lightly toasted and chopped (.5 cup)
- Also Needed: 9 x 13 pan

DIRECTIONS

1. Set the oven to 350° Fahrenheit. Lightly grease the baking pan and set aside.
2. Mix the semolina, flour, and baking powder in a mixing container.
3. Cream the butter with the sugar until light and fluffy using an electric mixer. With the mixer running, break in the egg yolks one by one. Continue mixing until the batter turns a light yellow color, and toss in the lemon zest and vanilla extract.
4. With the mixer on low speed, add the flour mixture in three batches alternating the sequence using the milk.
5. Beat the egg whites in a separate bowl with a pinch of salt until soft peaks form. Fold the egg whites into the batter until just blended. (Don't mix too much or you will "flatten" your egg whites.)
6. Pour the batter into the pan to bake for 45 minutes or until the cake is a golden color.
7. Prepare the syrup by adding the orange zest, sugar, and water to a saucepan. Wait for it to boil and set a timer for it to simmer for five minutes. Add the lemon juice and cool.
8. Cover the cake with the syrup while the cake is still warm. After the cake cools, sprinkle it as desired using the cinnamon, powdered sugar, or almonds.

Nutritions: Calories: 318 Protein: 5 grams Fat: 12 grams

6. GREEK STRAWBERRY FROZEN YOGURT

PREPARATION AND COOKINGTIME
2-4 HOURS

SERVING
16/1 QUART

INGREDIENTS

- **Fresh lemon juice (.25 cup)**
- **Salt (.125 tsp.)**
- **Sugar (1 cup)**
- **Vanilla (2 tsp.)**
- **2% plain Greek yogurt (3 cups)**
- **Sliced strawberries (1 cup)**
- **Also Needed: 1.5 to 2-quart ice cream maker**

DIRECTIONS

1. Whisk the vanilla, salt, lemon juice, yogurt, and sugar until it's creamy.
2. Place the mixture in the ice cream maker. Prepare the yogurt according to the manufacturer's instructions.
3. Toss in the sliced berries for the last minute of the cycle. Empty into a container and freeze for two to four hours before serving.
4. Let the ice cream sit out at room temperature for about 5 to 15 minutes before serving.

Nutritions: Calories: 86 Protein: 4 grams Fat: 1 gram

7. GRILLED ANGEL FOOD CAKE KEBABS

PREPARATION AND COOKINGTIME
20 MINUTES

SERVING
4 PEOPLE

INGREDIENTS

- **Whole strawberries (1 cup)**
- **Peach slices (1 cup)**
- **Angel food cake (1 cup of 1-inch cubes)**
- **Sugar (1 tbsp.)**
- **Ground cinnamon (.25 tsp.)**
- **Light white chocolate strawberry yogurt - ex. Yoplait (1 container - 6 oz.)**

DIRECTIONS

1. Heat a charcoal or gas grill.
2. Place the cake cubes, berries, and peaches alternately on the skewers.
3. Combine the cinnamon and sugar. Sprinkle over the kebabs.
4. Grill using the medium heat temperature setting.
5. Close the lid and cook about two minutes, turning once.
6. Serve with the yogurt when ready.

Nutritions: Protein: 2 grams Fat: 0 grams Calories: 100

8. GRILLED STONE FRUIT WITH WHIPPED RICOTTA

PREPARATION AND COOKINGTIME
20 MINUTES

SERVING
4 PEOPLE

INGREDIENTS

- **Apricots/plums - 8 or Peaches/ nectarines (4 - halved & pitted)**
- **Olive oil (2 tsp.)**
- **Whole-milk ricotta cheese (.75 cup)**
- **Honey (1 tbsp.)**
- **Freshly grated nutmeg (.25 tsp.)**
- **Optional Garnish: Mint sprigs (4)**

DIRECTIONS

1. Spray a grill pan or cold grill with a spritz of nonstick cooking spray. Heat up the grill using the medium heat temperature setting.
2. Place a large bowl in the fridge to chill.
3. Use oil to brush over the fruit and place onto the grill or pan with the cut side down. Cook for three to five minutes or until the grill marks appear on the skin.
4. Use tongs and turn the fruit over.
5. Cover with a lid for four to six minutes or until the skin is easily cut away. Set aside to cool.
6. Take the bowl out of the fridge and add the ricotta. Beat the ricotta using the high speed of an electric beater for about two minutes.
7. Pour in the honey and nutmeg. Continue cooking for another minute.
8. Divide the room temperature/ warm fruit into serving dishes.
9. Garnish with the ricotta concoction and a sprig of mint. Serve.

147

Nutritions: Calories: 176 Protein: 7 grams Fat: 9 grams

9. ITALIAN APPLE - OLIVE OIL CAKE

PREPARATION AND COOKINGTIME
1 HOUR 10 MIN

SERVING
12 PEOPLE

INGREDIENTS

- **Gala apples (2 large)**
- **Orange juice - for soaking apples**
- **All-purpose flour (3 cups)**
- **Ground cinnamon (.5 tsp.)**
- **Nutmeg (.5 tsp.)**
- **Baking powder (1 tsp.)**
- **Baking soda (1 tsp.)**
- **Sugar (1 cup)**
- **Olive oil (1 cup)**
- **Large eggs (2)**
- **Gold raisins (.66 cup)**
- **Confectioner's sugar - for dusting**
- **Also Needed: 9-inch baking pan**

DIRECTIONS

1. Peel and finely chop the apples. Drizzle the apples with just enough orange juice to prevent browning.
2. Soak the raisins in warm water for 15 minutes and drain well.
3. Sift the baking soda, flour, baking powder, cinnamon, and nutmeg. Set it to the side for now.
4. Pour the olive oil and sugar into the bowl of a stand mixer. Mix on the low setting for 2 minutes or until well combined.
5. Blend it while running, break in the eggs one at a time and continue mixing for 2 minutes. The mixture should increase in volume; it should be thick - not runny.
6. Combine all of the ingredients well Begin by making a hole in the center of the flour mixture and add in the olive and sugar mixture.
7. Remove the apples of any excess of juice and drain the raisins that have been soaking. Add them together with the batter, mixing well.
8. Prepare the baking pan with parchment paper. Scoop the batter into the pan and level it with the back of a wooden spoon.
9. Bake it for 45 minutes at a 350° Fahrenheit.
10. When ready, remove the cake from the parchment paper and place it into a serving dish. Dust with the confectioner's sugar. Heat dark honey to garnish the top.

Nutritions: Calories: 294 Protein: 5.3 grams Fat: 11 grams

10. STRAWBERRY RICOTTA PARFAITS

PREPARATION AND COOKINGTIME
30 MIN + 4 HOUR TO CHILL

SERVING
4 PEOPLE

INGREDIENTS

- **Fresh strawberries (1 lb.)**
- **Sugar (1 tsp.)**
- **Fresh mint (1 tbsp.)**
- **Part-skim ricotta cheese (15 oz.)**
- **Light agave nectar (3 tbsp.)**
- **Vanilla (.5 tsp.)**
- **Shredded lemon peel (.25 tsp.)**

DIRECTIONS

1. Combine the berries, mint, and sugar. Gently stir and marinate about 10 minutes until the berries soften.
2. Combine the ricotta, lemon peel, agave, and vanilla with an electric mixer for two minutes using the medium speed.
3. Assemble into chilled parfait glasses. Layer the ricotta mixture and top it off with the berries, alternating as desired.
4. Chill and cover for four hours.

Nutritions: Protein: 9 grams Fat: 6 grams Calories: 157

11. VANILLA GREEK YOGURT AFFOGATO

PREPARATION AND COOKINGTIME
10 MINUTES

SERVING
4 PEOPLE

INGREDIENTS

- **Vanilla Greek yogurt (24 oz.)**
- **Sugar (2 tsp.)**
- **Hot espresso (4 Shots) or (0.75 of a cup) strong brewed coffee**
- **Chopped - unsalted pistachios (4 tbsp.)**
- **Dark chocolate chips or shavings (4 tbsp.)**

DIRECTIONS

1. Spoon the yogurt into four tall chilled glasses.
2. Mix .5 teaspoon of sugar into each of the espresso shots.
3. Pour one shot of hot espresso or 1.5 ounces of coffee into each of the yogurt glasses.
4. Garnish each one off with the chocolate chips and pistachios before serving.

Nutritions: Calories: 270 Protein: 11 grams Fat: 10 grams

12. WATERMELON CUPS

PREPARATION AND COOKINGTIME
25 MINUTES

SERVING
16 PEOPLE

INGREDIENTS	DIRECTIONS

INGREDIENTS

- **Seedless watermelon cubes (16 - 1-inch)**
- **Finely chopped cucumber (.33 cup)**
- **Finely chopped red onion (5 tsp.)**
- **Minced fresh mint (2 tsp.)**
- **Lime juice (.5 to 1 tsp.)**
- **Freshly minced cilantro (2 tsp.)**

DIRECTIONS

1. Use a measuring spoon or a small melon baller to remove the center of each of the watermelon cubes. Leave a ¼-inch shell. Use the pulp another time.
2. In a small dish, mix the remaining fixings. Spoon into the watermelon cubes and serve.

Nutritions: Calories: 7 Protein: 0 grams Fat: 0 grams

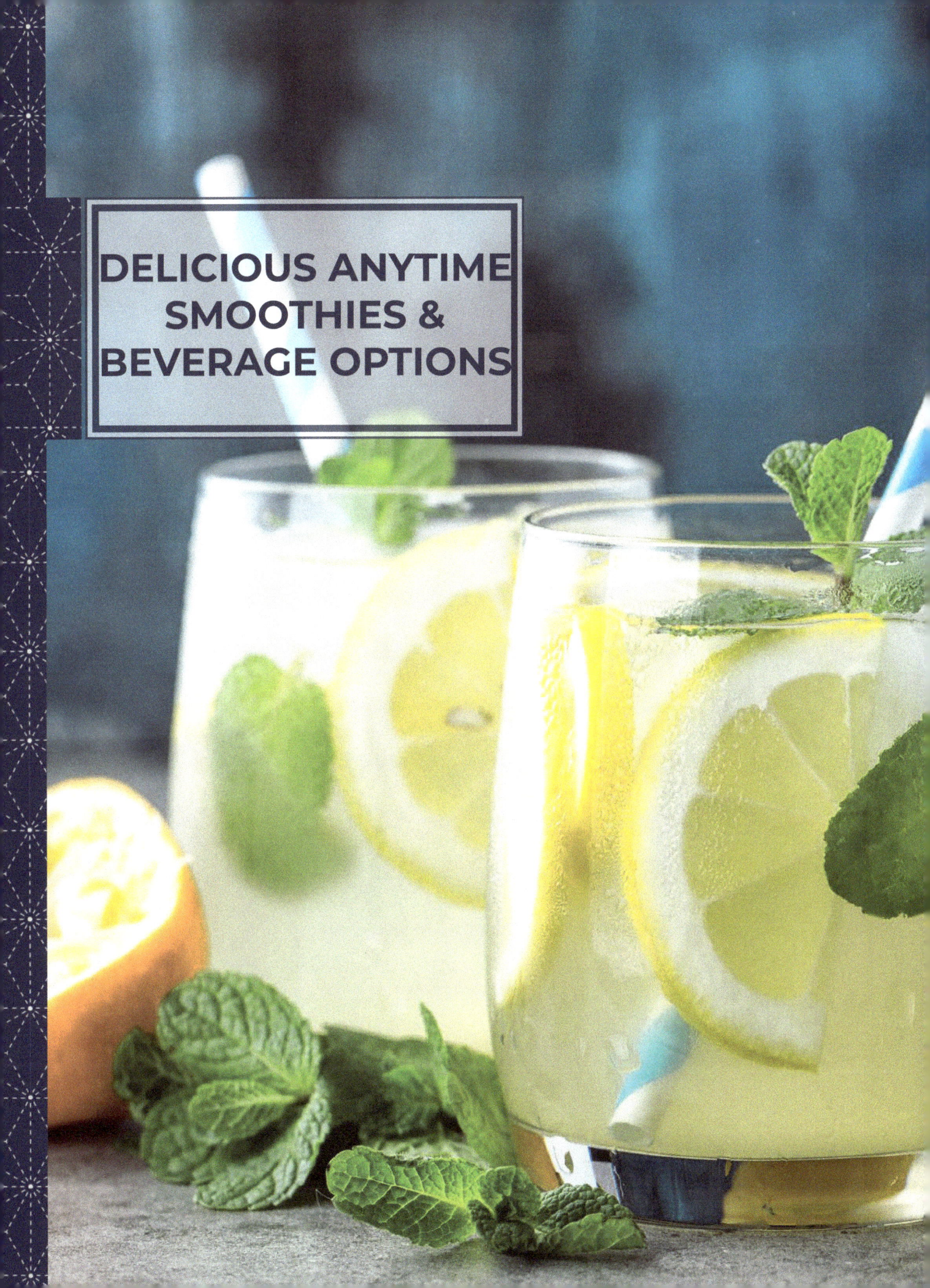

DELICIOUS ANYTIME SMOOTHIES & BEVERAGE OPTIONS

1. BLUEBERRY MARTINI CORDIALS

PREPARATION AND COOKINGTIME
20 MINUTES

SERVING
18 PEOPLE

INGREDIENTS

- **Blueberry yogurt (6 oz. container)**
- **Vanilla flavored vodka (.25 cup)**
- **Chocolate cordial cups (18)**
- **Blueberries (18)**
- **Also Needed: Toothpicks**
- **For the Garnish: Powdered sugar and mint sprigs**

DIRECTIONS

1. Whisk the vodka with the yogurt, mixing well.
2. Spoon it into the cups and place the berries onto the toothpicks. Place them in the cups.
3. Garnish with the mint sprig and powdered sugar before serving.

Nutritions: Calories: 60 Protein: 1 gram Fat: 2 grams

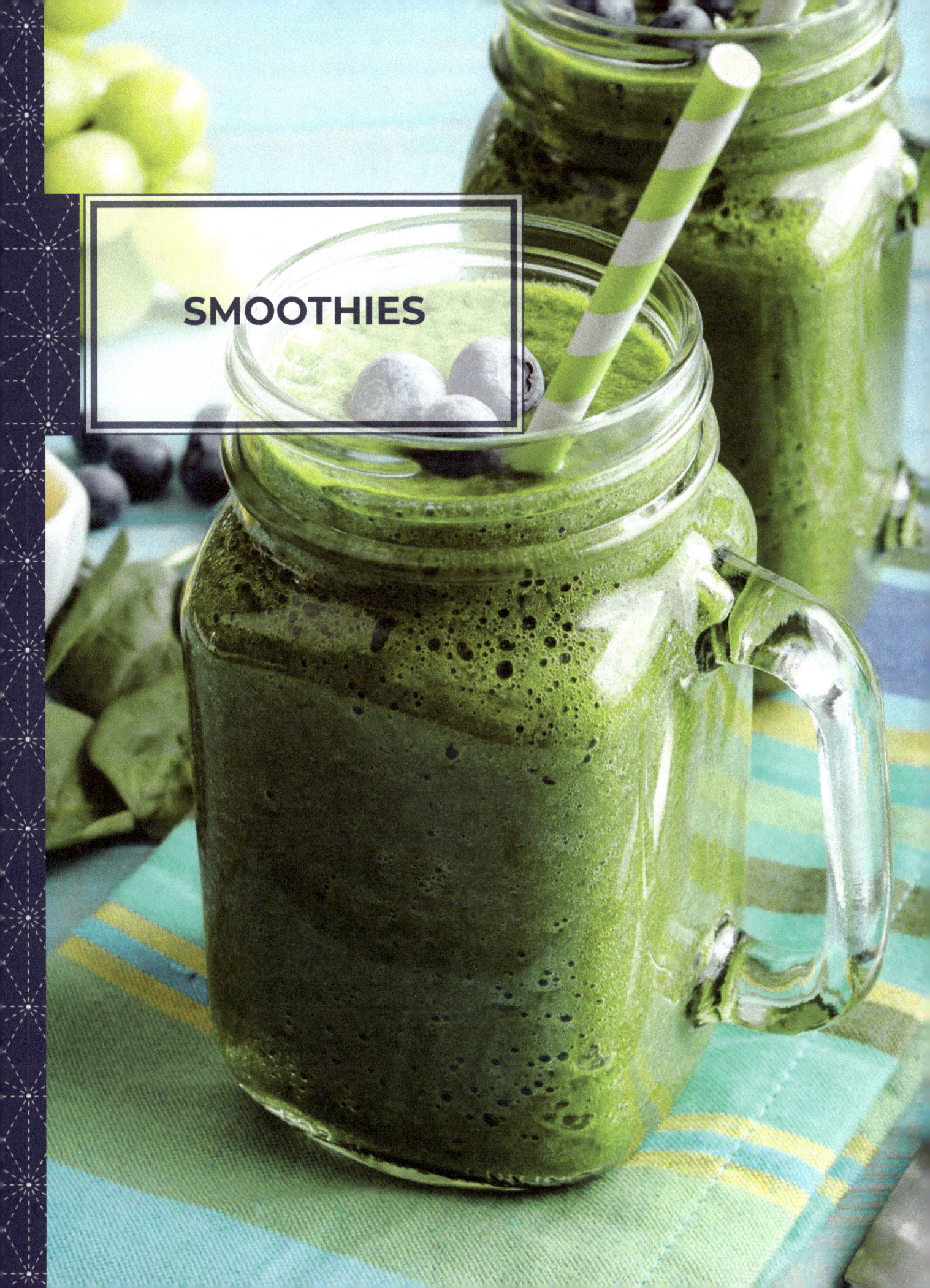

SMOOTHIES

2. ANTI-INFLAMMATORY BLUEBERRY SMOOTHIE

PREPARATION AND COOKINGTIME
5 MINUTES

SERVING
1 PEOPLE

INGREDIENTS

- **Almond milk (1 cup)**
- **Frozen banana (1)**
- **Frozen blueberries (⅔-1 cup)**
- **Leafy greens/spinach (2 handfuls)**
- **Almond butter (1 tbsp.)**
- **Cinnamon (.25 tsp.)**
- **Cayenne pepper (.125-.25 tsp.)**
- **Optional: Maca powder (1 tsp.)**

DIRECTIONS

1. Combine each of the fixings using a high-powered blender.
2. Mix thoroughly until creamy and serve in a chilled glass.

Nutritions: Calories: 340 Protein: 9 grams Fat: 13 grams

3. CHERRY - POMEGRANATE SMOOTHIE BOW - GLUTEN-FREE & VEGETARIAN

PREPARATION AND COOKINGTIME
5 MINUTES

SERVING
4 PEOPLE

INGREDIENTS

- **Frozen dark sweet cherries (16 oz. bag)**
- **2% Plain Greek yogurt (1.5 cups)**
- **Pomegranate juice (.75 cup)**
- **2% milk (.33 cup (+) more as needed)**
- **Ground cinnamon (.75 tsp.)**
- **Vanilla extract (1 tsp.)**
- **Fresh pomegranate seeds (.5 cup)**
- **Chopped pistachios (.5 cup)**
- **Ice cubes (6)**

DIRECTIONS

1. Chop the pistachios or purchase (arils) found in the produce section of the market. If you are using the whole fruit, remove the seeds underwater in a container so they will float to the top.
2. Add the fixings into a blender (ice, milk, cinnamon, vanilla, juice, yogurt, and cherries).
3. Pulse until it's creamy smooth. Use a little extra milk to thin the texture to get it to the desired consistency.
4. Pour the prepared smoothie into for dishes and top with two tablespoons of the chopped pistachios and two tablespoons of the seeds. Serve it immediately.

Nutritions: Calories: 212 Protein: 4 grams Fat: 7 grams

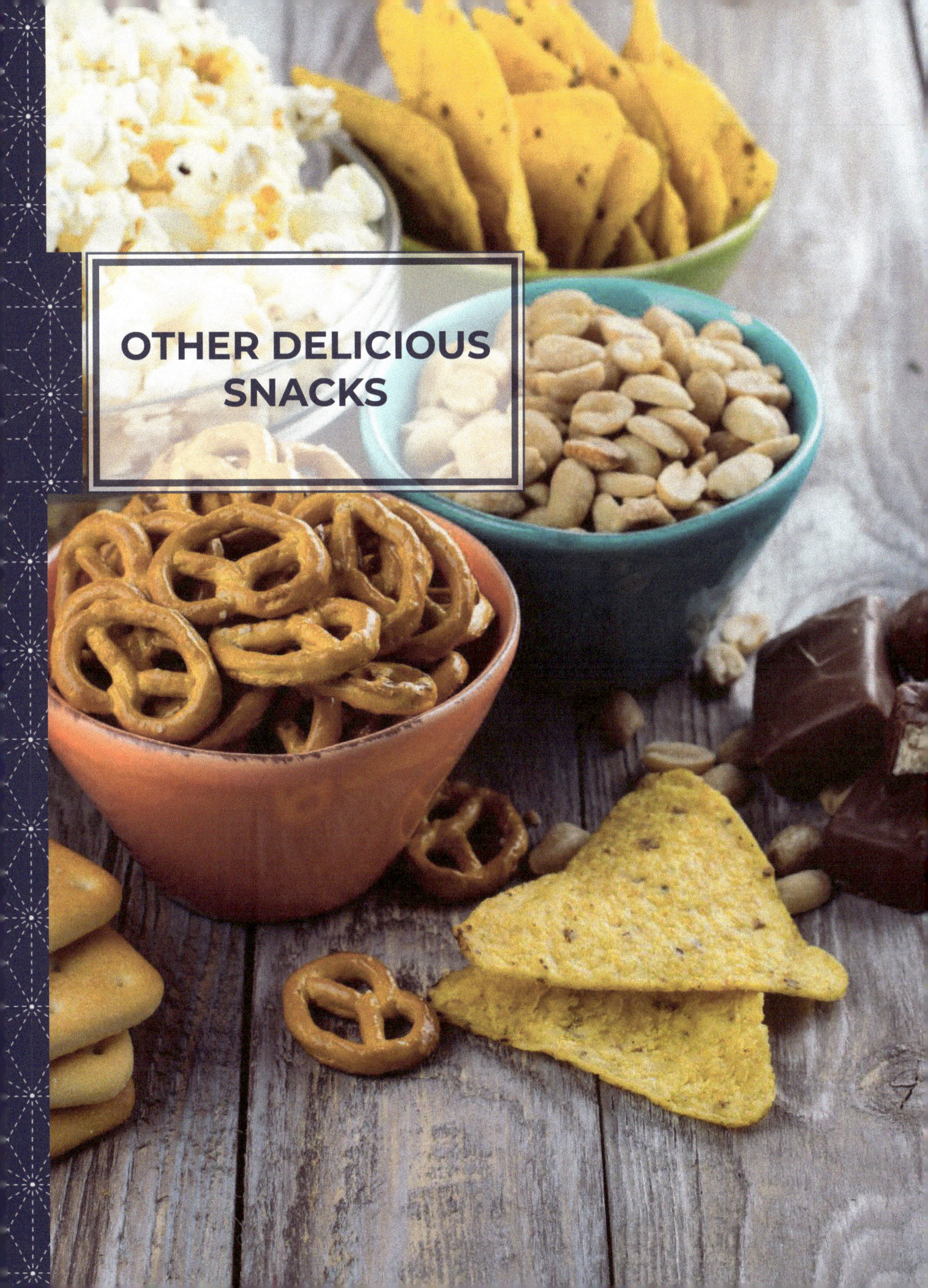

OTHER DELICIOUS SNACKS

1. ALMOND-STUFFED DATES

PREPARATION AND COOKINGTIME
5 MINUTES

SERVING
1 PEOPLE

INGREDIENTS

- **Whole almonds (2 salted)**
- **Pitted Medjool dates (2)**
- **Orange zest (.25 tsp.)**

DIRECTIONS

1. Stuff each one of the dates with one of the almonds.
2. Prepare the zest and roll each of the prepared dates through the mixture.
3. Serve as a snack, anytime.

Nutritions: Fat: 1.4 grams Calories: 149 Protein: 1.4 grams

2. DATE WRAPS

PREPARATION AND COOKINGTIME
10 MINUTES

SERVING
16 PEOPLE

INGREDIENTS

- **Whole pitted dates (16)**
- **Thinly sliced prosciutto (16 slices)**
- **Black pepper (as desired)**

DIRECTIONS

1. Wrap a slice of the prosciutto around each of the dates.
2. Serve with a shake of freshly ground black pepper.

Nutritions: Protein: 2.2 grams Fat: 0.8 grams Calories: 35

3. PISTACHIO NO-BAKE SNACK BARS

PREPARATION AND COOKINGTIME
10 MINUTES

SERVING
8 PEOPLE

INGREDIENTS

- **Pitted dates (20)**
- **Rolled old fashioned oats (1 cup)**
- **No-shell roasted & salted pistachios (1.25 cups)**
- **Unsweetened applesauce (.25 cup)**
- **Pistachio butter (2 tbsp.)**
- **Vanilla extract (1 tsp.)**
- **Also Needed: 8 by 8 baking dish and food processor fitted with a metal blade**

DIRECTIONS

1. Toss the dates to the processor. Process them for 30-45 seconds until pureed. Toss in the oats and pistachios. Pulse the mixture in 15-second intervals for two to three times until a crumbly, coarse consistency is achieved.
2. Pour the applesauce, pistachio butter, and vanilla extract into the processor and pulse 20-30 seconds until dough is slightly sticky.
3. Line the pan with parchment baking paper.
4. Use a spatula to transfer the dough from the processor and pour it into the pan. Press down firmly to evenly distribute the dough using another piece of parchment paper.
5. Lift the paper and place evenly with the remaining 1/4 cup of no-shell pistachios - onto the top of the dough.
6. Pop the pan in the freezer with parchment paper over the top and freeze for at least one hour before slicing.
7. Slice it into eight bars and keep them in the fridge for up to a week.
8. Note: To make pistachio butter, take one cup 'no-shell' pistachios and place in a food processor with one teaspoon vanilla extract. Process for three to four minutes, scraping down the sides as needed, until smooth.

Nutritions: Calories: 220 Protein: 6 grams Fat: 12 grams

4. QUINOA GRANOLA

PREPARATION AND COOKINGTIME
30 MINUTES

SERVING
7 PEOPLE

INGREDIENTS

- **Old-fashioned rolled oats (1 cup)**
- **Uncooked Bob's Red Mill White Quinoa or your choice (.5 cup)**
- **Raw almonds (2 cups roughly chopped)**
- **Coconut sugar/organic brown sugar (1 tbsp.)**
- **Coconut oil (3.5 tbsp.)**
- **Sea salt (1 pinch)**
- **Maple syrup or agave nectar (.25 cup)**

DIRECTIONS

1. Heat the oven to reach 340° Fahrenheit.
2. Combine the almonds, quinoa, oats, salt, and coconut sugar in a large mixing container. Shake lightly to blend.
3. Pour the maple syrup and coconut oil into a saucepan. Warm it up using medium heat for two to three minutes. Whisk frequently until the two are thoroughly combined. Mix in with the dry fixings and the oats and nuts until covered. Arrange on a cookie sheet in an even layer.
4. Bake for 20 minutes.
5. Transfer from the oven and stir/toss the granola. Put the opposite end of the pan back into the oven and bake 5 to 10 more minutes.
6. Cool completely before serving.

Nutritions: Calories: 332 Protein: 9 grams Fat: 21 grams

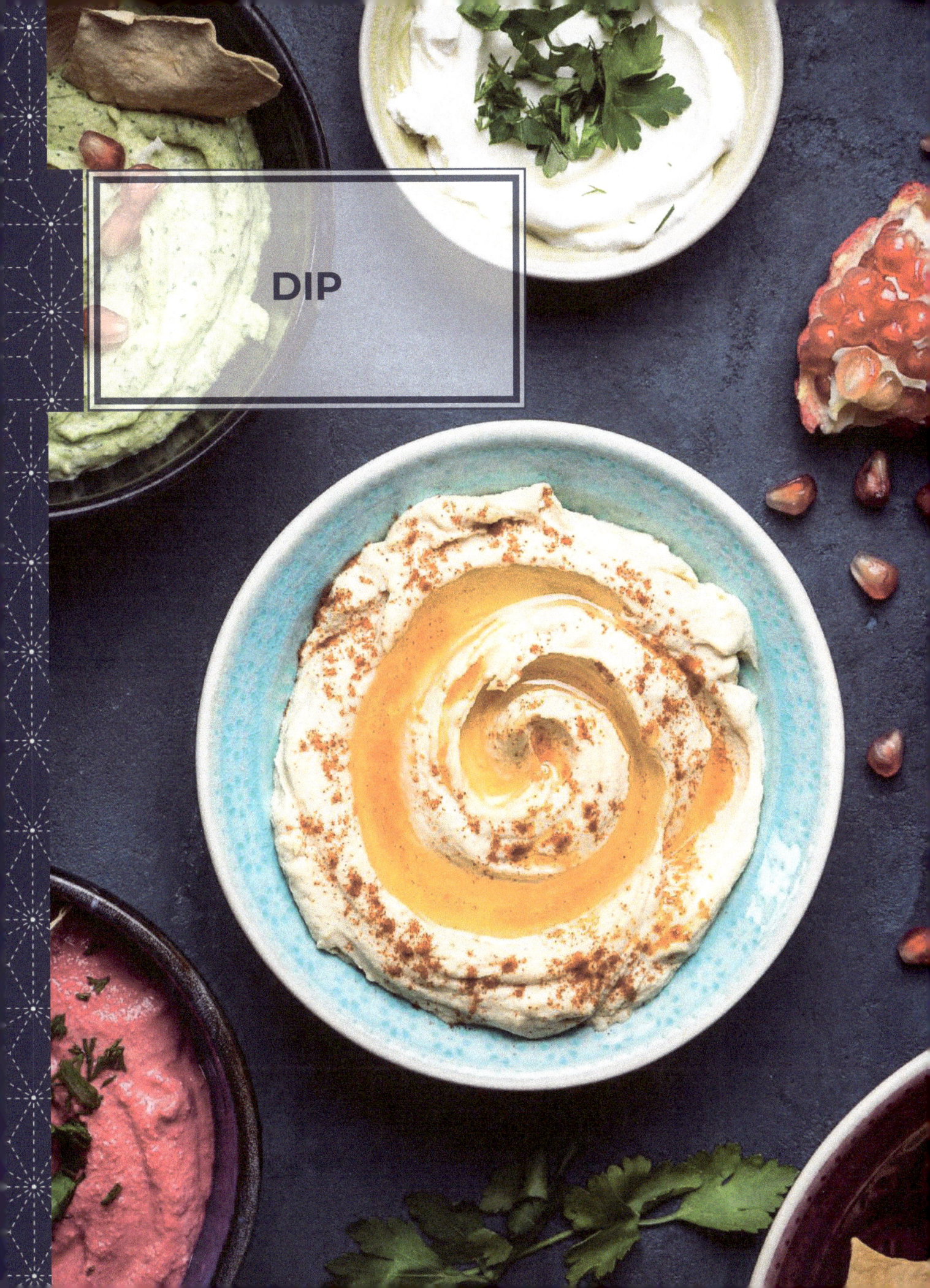

DIP

1. GARLIC GARBANZO BEAN SPREAD

PREPARATION AND COOKINGTIME
MINUTES

SERVING
1.5 CUPS

INGREDIENTS

- **Chickpeas or garbanzo beans (15 oz. can)**
- **Olive oil (.5 cup)**
- **Green onion (1-3 pieces)**
- **Lemon juice (1 tbsp.)**
- **Garlic cloves (1-2 peeled)**
- **Salt (.25 tsp.)**
- **Freshly minced parsley (2 tbsp.)**
- **Baked pita chips and assorted fresh veggies (add the carbs)**
- **Also Needed: Food Processor**

DIRECTIONS

1. Combine the chickpeas or garbanzo beans, oil, parsley, lemon juice, garlic, salt, and green onion.
2. Add the ingredients into the blender and process until mixed.
3. Empty into a dish and refrigerate until ready to serve.
4. Enjoy with the pita chips and veggies.

Nutritions: Calories: 114 per 2 tbsp. Serving Protein: 1 gram Fat: 10 grams

2. SPICY SWEET ROASTED RED PEPPER HUMMUS

PREPARATION AND COOKINGTIME
5 MINUTES

SERVING
8 PEOPLE

INGREDIENTS

- **Garbanzo beans - drained (15 oz. can)**
- **Lemon juice (3 tbsp.)**
- **Roasted red peppers (4 oz. jar)**
- **Tahini (1.5 tbsp.)**
- **Minced garlic (1 clove)**
- **Cayenne pepper (.5 tsp.)**
- **Salt (.25 tsp.)**
- **Ground cumin (.5 tsp.)**
- **Chopped fresh parsley (1 tbsp.)**

DIRECTIONS

1. Prepare all of the fixings in a food processor/blender.
2. When fluffy and smooth, add it to a serving dish for at least one hour. Return the hummus to room temperature when it is time to serve.

Nutritions: Protein: 2.5 grams Fat: 2.2 grams Calories: 64

9.
7-DAY MEAL PLAN

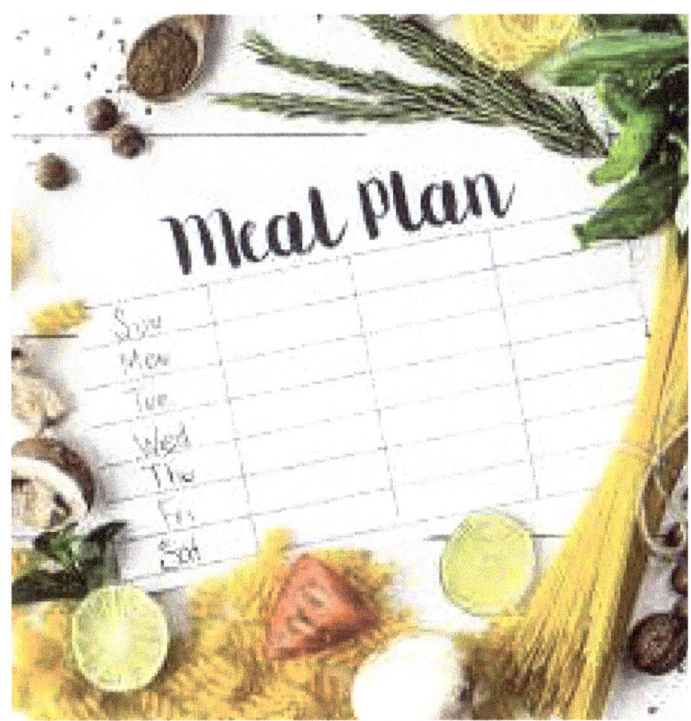

This type of plan has long been hailed as the 'gold standard' of healthy diets. It cannot be accurately defined in a single sentence because it is used throughout the entire coastlines of the Mediterranean Sea, serving more than 18 countries. There are food patterns that emerge, so in a 'nut-shell,' this plan is the best way to reap the benefits.

Day 1:

Breakfast: Zucchini Egg White Frittata - 137

Snack: Cherry - Pomegranate Smoothie Bow - Gluten-Free & Vegetarian - 212

Lunch: Slow-Cooked Mediterranean Roasted Turkey Breast - 333

Dinner: Baked Salmon With Dill - 251

Dessert: Italian Apple - Olive Oil Cake - 294

Day 2:

Breakfast: Feta - Avocado & Mashed Chickpea Toast - 337

Snack: Almond-Stuffed Dates - 149

Lunch: Niçoise-Style Tuna Salad With Olives & White Beans - 548

Dinner: Mixed Spice Burgers - 231

Dessert: Herb-Crusted Halibut - 273

Day 3:

Breakfast: Marinara Eggs With Parsley - Gluten-Free - 122

Snack: Greek Strawberry Frozen Yogurt - 86

Lunch: Lemon Chicken Skewers - 219

Dinner: Tilapia With Avocado & Red Onion - 200

Dessert: Blueberry Martini Cordials - 60/Chocolate Almond Butter Fruit Dip - 115

Day 4:

Breakfast: Nutty Orange Polenta - 234

Snack: Watermelon Cups - 7

Lunch: Feta Chicken Burgers - 356

Dinner: Marinated Tuna Steak - 200

Dessert: Chilled Dark Chocolate Fruit Kebabs - 254

Day 5:

Breakfast: Pumpkin Pancakes - 278

Snack: Italian Celery & Orange Salad - Gluten-Free - 65

Lunch: Greek Lentil Soup - 357

Dinner: Pan-Seared Salmon - 271

Dessert: Grilled Stone Fruit With Whipped Ricotta - 176

Day 6:

Breakfast: Scrambled Eggs With Roasted Peppers & Goat Cheese - Gluten-Free - 201

Snack: Date Wraps - 35

Lunch: Tomato Salad - Grilled Halloumi & Herbs - 196

Dinner: Mediterranean Flounder - 282

Dessert: Avocado - Chocolate Pudding With Hazelnuts & Sea Salt - 295

Day 7:

Breakfast: 5-Minute Heirloom Tomato & Cucumber Toast - 177

Snack: Quinoa Granola -332

Lunch: Honey Lime Fruit Salad - 115

Dinner: Chicken Thighs With Shallots In Red Wine Vinegar - 353.5

Dessert: Strawberry Ricotta Parfaits - 157

How to Plan the Diet Meal Plan & the Shopping List

Make Extra-virgin olive oil your main fat. This bit of 'liquid gold' will be your press friend, whether you want to generously apply it to your fish or veggies before grilling or roasting. You can make simple Vinaigrette for your salad or use a drizzle over your bean soups, potatoes, or steamed veggies to bring out the natural flavors.

Eat Plenty of Fish: This is one that cannot be mentioned often enough and is called the 'Eskimo factor.' The Eskimos loaded up on seal and whale meat, which meant they had a diet low in complex carbohydrates, vegetables, and fruits.

On the other hand, they consumed about 15 grams (about ½ ounce) of fish oil daily, making it the centerpiece of the diet plan rich in marine omega-3 polyunsaturated fatty acids, which are very heart-healthy. Try some albacore tuna packed in water over your greens at lunch with some olive oil vinaigrette. If you are eating out at your favorite steak house, ask for a tuna or salmon steak making sure it is grilled and only has a squeeze of lemon.

Eat plenty of whole grains: You can enjoy natural and fresh foods, and leave the refined and process ones on the grocer's shelf. You want to aim for at least three servings of whole grains daily. Try some of these for a change of pace:

- Make a bowl of tasty oatmeal for breakfast for most of the week. Choose the steel-cut version since they contain the highest levels of beta-glucan. You can reheat it in just a few minutes.

- Have some popcorn and give it a spray of some olive oil and a sprinkle of brown sugar for a sweet treat or a salty one try some parmesan cheese.

- Be sure to choose 100% whole grain muffins, bagels, and loaves of bread for your sandwiches.

Have some colorful veggies and greens for lunch and dinner daily. You know what that includes, those crunchy flashy colored bell peppers or some juicy red tomatoes with some thick dark green spinach. This type of eating will assist in keeping your arteries clean and healthy. Here are a few simple ways to enlist the greens into your diet plan even with a busy lifestyle:

- Toss in a few of your favorite bagged, pre-washed, and pre-chopped veggies on a baking sheet with a bit of foil. Drizzle some oil on them and roast them for at least thirty minutes at 425° Fahrenheit.

-

- Whether you are at home or dining out, have a healthy, dark green salad for lunch or dinner using some fresh lemon juice, or vinegar, or some (yes, you guessed it) olive oil.

Incorporate some lentils or other types of legumes. There is no need to spend a lot of money on these yummy nutritional legumes because you can purchase them for 'pennies on a dollar.' The legumes can be found in many colors, sizes, and shapes, but no matter how you find them, they are an excellent choice for your diet plan.

Some of the legumes include peas, lupins, beans, or chickpeas, which are part of the culinary culture of the diet plan basis. Each of these huge nutritional selections offers heart-healthy Ingredients, including plant protein, fiber, vitamins, antioxidants, iron, and minerals.

Try some of these suggestions to break up the monotony of a regular day:

- Sprinkle some legumes such as kidney beans or chickpeas on your salad (after you rinse and drain them).

- Dip raw veggies into some hummus.

- Eat legume-based soups such as black bean, minestrone, split pea, lentil, or Pasta e Fagioli (pasta and beans).

- Snack on some mouth-watering edamame (soybeans). This can be found frozen in the supermarket or as an appetizer on one of your outings to a Japanese restaurant.

Enjoy some walnuts. Walnuts will provide you with alpha-linolenic acid (ALA), which will provide you with additional omega-3s. Try to add some of these to your snack routine:

- For a sweet snack, throw a few in the oven with a bit of brown sugar.

- Sprinkle some nuts on your green salads

- Keep a bag of shelled nuts on the countertop for a quick and healthy snack.

- Sprinkle some over some fat-free Greek yogurt with a drizzle of honey.

Have some dark chocolate: Scientific evidence has proven deep-dark chocolate is a visible link with the phenomenal health benefits, including your heart, especially! Before you indulge, think of the "real" cocoa and not just a solid chocolate bar. Unsweetened cocoa powder is low in fat, calories, and sugar.

Top off your day with a delicious cup of hot chocolate. Use a small amount of sweetener or sugar substitute with two heaping teaspoonfuls of natural unsweetened cocoa powder and soy milk.

Indulge in some wine for dinner: Wine is also a provider of antioxidant polyphenols, which makes the wine part of a plan to help reduce the risk of heart attacks. Choose the red instead of the white because it contains more of the beneficial antioxidants. But remember ladies; just one—and gents you can have two.

Incorporate these items into your basic meal plan, but be sure you always count all calories consumed every day to achieve the best results.

Use Meal Prep Techniques for Those Busy Schedules

If you have a busy lifestyle and don't have the time to prepare a full-course meal every night, why not choose a day to prepare different foods to use throughout the week? Meal prep might seem a bit challenging at first but just remember – you don't need to prep all of your meals at one time. You can begin with the meats one evening, and veggies the next; it's all up to you!

Ask A Few Simple Questions: Do you want to prepare all of the chicken, pork, or other meal selections one night and the veggies the next night? Or: Do you want to cook each meal individually but in bulk? Either way works.

Select A Non-Busy Preparation Day: Choose a time when you won't have

any interruptions.

Purchase Appropriate Containers: These are some guidelines for those:

- Mason Jars – Pint or quart-sized
- Ziploc-type freezer bags
- Rubbermaid Stackable
- Glad Containers
- Freezer Safe
- Microwavable
- BPA-Free
- Reusable
- Stackable

Label the Containers: There are some other things you have to consider when freezing your meals. You should always label your container with the date that you put it in the freezer. You also need to double-check that your bottles, jars, or bags are each sealed tightly. If your containers aren't air-tight, your food will become freezer burnt and need to be trashed.

By using meal prep, you will find you can always have a healthy choice for your Mediterranean style eating. Start small with your prepping and see how it goes.

CONCLUSION

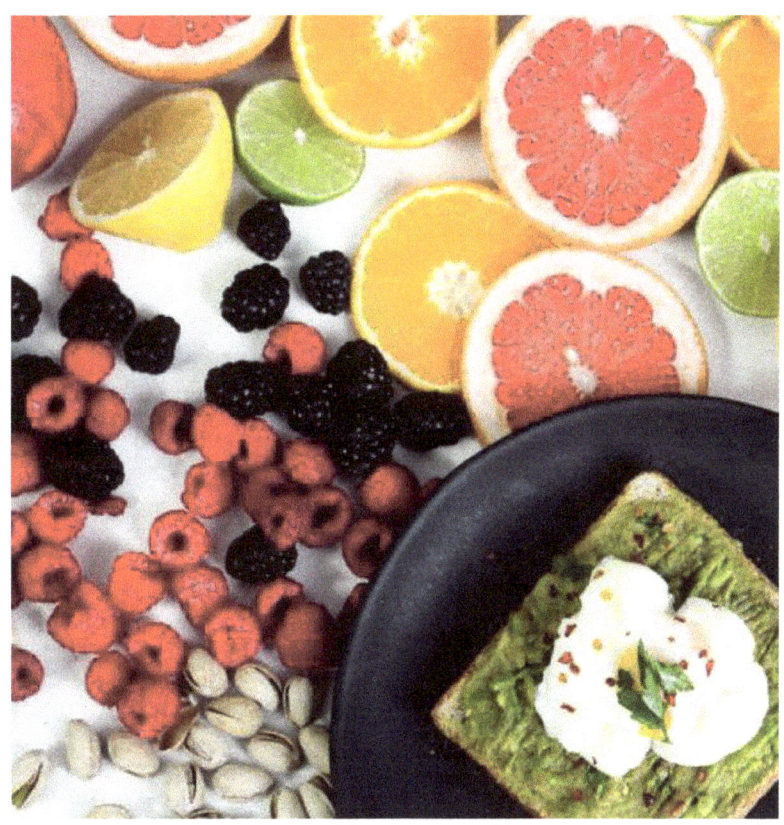

Thank you for making it through to the end of Mediterranean Diet, let's hope it was informative provided you with all of the tools you need to achieve your goals, whatever they may be. You have the basic meal plan calculated for seven days, but you will find there is not a lot of hard to find Ingredients included in the simple Mediterranean diet plan.

The next step is to understand the Mediterranean food pyramid fully. The basic guidelines for your daily allowances are included:

- 3 Servings: Fruit - Dairy Products

- 6 Servings: Vegetables

- 8 Servings: Non-refined products and cereals (brown rice, whole grain bread, etc.)

Unlimited: Water, Water, and More Water!

Your Weekly Allowance:

- 3 Servings: Eggs - Potatoes - Sweets

- 3-4 Servings: Nuts, Olives, Pulses

- 7-14 tbsp.: Olive oil

- 4 Servings: Legumes & Poultry

- 5-6 Servings: Fish

Your Monthly Allowance:

- 4 Servings: Red meat

One of the easiest ways to remain on your Mediterranean diet while dining out is to take the edge off of your hunger before you leave home, especially if you are really hungry. Enjoy a high-protein and low-calorie snack such as yogurt to help you feel full, which will help you from overeating. Eliminate the sugary sweet drinks. Water cannot be stressed enough while you are attempting to drop the pounds since it helps keep you hydrated and steers the hunger away.

Avoid Anything Fried: Ask your waiter/waitress for your food to be prepared specifically without any frying.

About Appetizers: Remove the temptation and ask the waiter/waitress not to bring a bread-and-butter basket to the table. If you are hungry, you may be tempted to eat more than you should. Avoid fried appetizers. Stick with some steamed fish or shellfish, mixed salads, broth-based soups, or grilled veggies. Share your appetizer, so that you will have a smaller portion.

About the Entree: Choose from fish, lean pork (center-cut or tenderloin), and poultry or vegetarian choices. If you are bound for red meat, select the leaner cuts such as flank, sirloin, filet mignon, or a tenderloin. You might also want to consider the beef will have a higher calorie and higher fat count. Ask for substitutes for items including mashed potatoes, macaroni salad, potato salad, coleslaw, or French fries. Instead, choose a side salad, steamed rice, baked potato, or steamed veggies.

Use caution with sauces. Avoid sauces with cream, cheese, oil, or butter. Request that the sauces be served in a separate container, so you can add what is allowed. Use your fork to dip the sauce to limit the temptation of over-indulging.

Enjoy your meal, and eat slowly. Ask to have the plate removed when you feel full. Eat only half of the portion or share it with a friend. You can always ask for a 'to-go bag' and enjoy the leftovers later. It will be an excellent lunch for tomorrow. You can also ask for half of the meal to be held in the kitchen until you are through with your meal. Once again, just remove the temptation!

About Dessert: Have a cup of coffee, cappuccino, or some herbal tea with a sugar substitute or no sugar with some skim milk. Order a dessert for everyone at the table to enjoy. Order some berries or mixed fruit.

Savor A Delicious Glass Of Wine: Red wine has certain properties that have shown are beneficial for heart health. The cardio-protection provided by red wine is attributed to the antioxidants in the skin of the grapes, which help lower your risk of heart disease by increasing good cholesterol, lowering bad cholesterol, and reducing blood clotting.

Even though it is believed that red wine is part of your healthy lifestyle, you must be cautious. The daily recommended intake for women is just (1) 4-oz. glass. For men, you can consume (2) 4-oz. glasses.

Slow Down: Try eating slower and chewing your food more thoroughly. Put your utensils down between mouthfuls to help slow you down. It will also give you time for satiety to kick in.

Finally, if you found this book useful in any way, a review on Amazon is always appreciated!

Index of Recipes

For your meal planning convenience, each of the recipes has the calorie counts listed!

Chapter 1: Mediterranean Breakfast Dishes

Chapter 2: Mediterranean Lunchtime & Dinner Salad & Side Favorites

- Herb Antipasto Pasta Salad Platter - 543
- Honey Lime Fruit Salad - 115
- Insalata Caprese II Salad - 311
- Italian Celery & Orange Salad - Gluten-Free - 65
- Mediterranean Pasta Salad - 259
- Salad In A Sandwich - 462
- Shrimp Orzo Salad - Mediterranean -Style - 397
- 3-Ingredient Mediterranean Salad - 104
- Tomato Salad - Grilled Halloumi & Herbs - 196
- Tuna Antipasto Salad - 306
- Turkish Orange Salad With Mediterranean Dressing - 186

Favorite Side Dishes & Tapas

- Avocado & Tuna Tapas - 194
- Cannellini Bean Lettuce Wraps - 235
- Easy Farfalle with Fresh Tomatoes - 212.5
- Fried Rice With Spinach - Peppers & Artichokes - 244
- Gigantes (Greek Lima Beans) - 449
- Gluten-Free Spanish Rice - 170
- Greek Baked Zucchini & Potatoes - Briam - 534
- Green Beans & Feta - 80
- Kale - Mediterranean-Style - 91
- Mediterranean Endive Boats - 715
- Mediterranean Nachos - 170
- Mediterranean Potatoes - 207.8
- Melitzanes Imam/Greek Eggplant Dish - 314
- Red Mediterranean Potato Salad - 60

Chapter 6: Mediterranean Dinner Pork Options

Pork Favorites:

Lamb Favorites

Chapter 7: Mediterranean Bread - Flatbread & Pizzas

Meal Choices

Mediterranean Pizza

Chapter 8: Desserts - Fruity Treats & More

- Greek Semolina Cake With Orange Syrup - Revani - 318
- Greek Strawberry Frozen Yogurt - 86
- Grilled Angel Food Cake Kebabs - 100
- Grilled Stone Fruit With Whipped Ricotta - 176
- Italian Apple - Olive Oil Cake - 294
- Strawberry Ricotta Parfaits - 157
- Vanilla Greek Yogurt Affogato - 270
- Watermelon Cups - 7

Delicious Anytime Smoothies & Beverage Options

- Blueberry Martini Cordials - 60

Smoothies

- Anti-Inflammatory Blueberry Smoothie - 340
- Cherry - Pomegranate Smoothie Bow - Gluten-Free & Vegetarian - 212

Other Delicious Snacks

- Almond-Stuffed Dates - 149
- Date Wraps - 35
- Pistachio No-Bake Snack Bars - 220
- Quinoa Granola -332

Dips

- Garlic Garbanzo Bean Spread - 114
- Spicy Sweet Roasted Red Pepper Hummus - 64

CPSIA information can be obtained
at www.ICGtesting.com
Printed in the USA
LVHW071739081220
673564LV00013B/161